THE New
CABBAGE
SOUP
DIET

The New
CABBAGE
SOUP
DIET

Revised and Updated Edition

MARGARET DANBROT

A Lynn Sonberg Book

St. Martin's Paperbacks

THE NEW CABBAGE SOUP DIET

Copyright © 1997, 2004 by Lynn Sonberg Book Associates.

ISBN: 0-312-99240-8
EAN: 80312-99240-8

Printed in the United States of America

St. Martin's Press Paperbacks edition / February 1997
St. Martin's Press Paperbacks revised edition / February 2004

St. Martin's Paperbacks are published by St. Martin's Press, 175 Fifth Avenue, New York, NY 10010.

20   19   18   17   16   15   14   13

IMPORTANT NOTE TO READERS

The reader should consult his or her physician before beginning this or any other diet. Consulting one's physician is particularly important if one is suffering from any illness or on any medication. All readers, however, should speak with their doctors before starting this diet to be sure it is appropriate for them.

The New Cabbage Soup Diet is not appropriate for long-term use. It is not intended as a substitute for good long-term eating habits. The diet may be used for up to a week, but after a week the reader should switch to a normal nutritionally balanced diet for at least two weeks before returning to the New Cabbage Soup Diet. The reader should not use the New Cabbage Soup Diet too frequently even with two-week or longer intervals in between uses.

Under no circumstances is the diet appropriate for children or adolescents.

CONTENTS

CHAPTER 1

The Excitement Continues

Back in 1997, *The New Cabbage Soup Diet* hit the bookstores. Talk about success! Since then thousands of men and women have lost up to ten pounds in seven days with this unique food plan—easily, safely, and without ever feeling hungry.

They used the New Cabbage Soup Diet to get back to feeling trim after holiday or vacation bingeing.

They used it to crash off pounds before bathing suit season or to quickly lose the extra inches that were spoiling the fit of a favorite outfit.

They used it to slim down just enough to look their best for a big event.

Other dieters—those who wanted and needed to lose large amounts of weight—used the New Cabbage Soup Diet, too. Some used it to jump-start the weight-loss process before embarking on a more moderate, well-balanced weight-loss regimen.

Or they used it to get back into weight-loss mode after hitting a diet plateau.

They even used it to blitz off the last few stubborn pounds, the ones that stood between them and their weight-loss goal.

Here, in this revised edition of *The New Cabbage Soup Diet*, you will find all the information that made the original New Cabbage Soup Diet a hit with dieters across the United

States and elsewhere—complete with food plans, nutrition updates, recipe ideas, step-by-step guidelines, rules to lose by, tips for better results. And, because achieving your weight-loss goal will depend on cultivating a positive "losing" attitude, you will also find suggestions to help you prime your mind for success.

This revised edition contains all that and more, including new information that will help make losing the weight you want to lose even easier.

You'll hear from successful dieters, discover how they dealt with problems, find out what worked for them and what didn't, learn from their triumphs and mistakes.

You'll find out about the physical and psychological benefits of exercise—including how it can help you lose pounds and keep them off, how to custom-tailor an exercise program that fits your lifestyle, how to ease into it, and how to make it fun.

And you'll find out how to use New Cabbage Soup Diet principles and recipes to maintain your weight once you've achieved your goal.

Ready? Then let's begin!

BEGINNING AT THE BEGINNING

First, congratulations are in order! You've chosen the one diet book that will help you change your life forever. Within these pages you will discover the secret to getting a huge jump-start on significant weight loss—ten pounds or even more in a week!—as well as a plan for conquering all the diet challenges you may encounter on your way to reaching your ideal weight. That jump-start and that plan are what the New Cabbage Soup Diet is all about.

As you will soon see, the Cabbage Soup Diet is unlike any diet you've ever tried. In fact, it is so extraordinary that in telling you all about it, we're going to deviate from the classic diet book formula.

For instance, most diet books begin with a lengthy pep

talk to motivate the dieter and generate enthusiasm for the diet. There are dozens of reasons to feel upbeat and enthusiastic about the Cabbage Soup Diet: It's unique. (In fact, it's in a class by itself, unlike any weight-loss plan you've heard or read about.) It's different in structure, ingredients, and procedure, and these differences help make it super-effective at moving your body into quick weight-loss mode. It's easy to follow. It keeps you feeling full and satisfied all day every day you use it. And it enables you to lose more weight than you ever thought possible in the short time you are on it. It even comes in two versions: a seven-day plan and a three-day blitz plan. And, of course, there is also a Cabbage Soup Maintenance Plan.

In the pages to come you will learn what makes the New Cabbage Soup Diet the quick weight-loss phenomenon it is, as well as how to follow it. But for now, let's take a look at what we know and don't know about its background.

THE SACRED HEART DIET—NOT

The Cabbage Soup Diet has been one of the most talked about and written about weight-loss plans of the last few years. (If you look it up on the Internet, you'll find hundreds of articles about the diet and thousands of mentions.) Its fame among dieters grew without an army of promoters banging the drums for it, without medical endorsements, and until the original *New Cabbage Soup Diet* was published, without even a book explaining what it's all about.

How did the excitement begin? Word of mouth. News of this easy, effective plan for losing weight spread from one enthusiastic dieter eager to share his or her weight-loss success to the next—face-to-face, by phone, by fax, and on the Internet. Soon the Cabbage Soup Diet was being mentioned everywhere, in such newspapers as the *Washington Post* and the *New York Times*, in magazines like *Cosmopolitan*, and on local and national television. You've probably heard or read about this diet yourself, and perhaps the excitement you felt then even motivated you to buy this book!

Actually, there are a number of different Cabbage Soup Diets circulating out there. Most of these versions are called simply the "Cabbage Soup Diet." But some go by other names, such as the "Fat Burning Soup Diet" and the "T-J Miracle Soup Diet." It has also been called the "Rochester Diet," the "New Mayo Clinic Diet," and, most commonly, the "Sacred Heart Hospital Diet."

It is important to be clear right away that no Sacred Heart Hospital (there are many—at least one in almost every area of the country) uses or recommends a diet based on cabbage soup, and neither does the Mayo Clinic. In fact, it is highly unlikely that the diet came from any hospital or medical center. Why do we say this?

SPEED—THE CRITICAL DIFFERENCE

The Cabbage Soup Diet gives you quick results. Diets recommended by major medical institutions work slowly, producing a one- to two-pound weight loss in a week or ten days. These diets are good, nutritionally sound programs. The slowness factor is built in, partly to help dieters change their food habits over time. The thinking is that if we follow one of these moderate, balanced food plans long enough, we will gradually learn to make healthier food choices and incorporate the principles of good nutrition into our lives. When that happens, we may be able to maintain a desirable weight over the months and years.

Developing healthful eating habits is a worthwhile goal, one we should all strive to achieve, and later on in this book you will learn the basic principles of good nutrition. But unfortunately, lack of early signs of success is also a major drawback of those same moderate, balanced programs. Most of us start a diet wanting and hoping to see tangible results fairly quickly. Discouragement often sets in when, after a week or ten days of dieting, the bathroom scale registers a loss of just a pound or so. And for too many of us, discouragement leads to abandonment of the slow but steady, moderate and well-balanced diet. We may throw up our hands and say, "What's the use? At this rate I'll *never* get rid of the pounds I want to lose."

It's important to emphasize that the sensible but slow-working diets endorsed by the nutrition establishment are models of good nutrition and excellent for the long haul, when you want and need to lose forty, fifty, sixty pounds, or more. But no matter who endorses it, a slow-working diet of any kind is among the least effective weight-loss plans if it turns you off at the beginning, when you are most eager to see signs of progress, and when quick weight loss, momentum, and motivation matter most.

The Cabbage Soup Diet addresses the classic diet problem in which impatience, frustration, and discouragement war against achieving substantial results. In offering quick weight loss, it provides the momentum and motivation you need to keep going.

Use the Cabbage Soup Diet for seven days to experience the gratification of quick weight loss. Then stop, use the Cabbage Soup Maintenance plan for two weeks or more, then go back to the diet again.

Or use this remarkable weight-loss plan for seven days, be inspired by the almost immediate results you've achieved as the diet propels you toward your goal, then switch to a more moderate and balanced long-term plan.

In either case, the heightened confidence and motivation you get from a week of incredible diet success will help keep you on track and moving forward.

MYSTERY DIET? MAYBE . . .

The question remains: If the Cabbage Soup Diet wasn't developed by a major medical institution, where did it come from? We can only guess. Perhaps it was conceived by a lone doctor somewhere, a doctor who wanted to help motivate certain patients to lose weight and came up with a cabbage soup–based diet that would reward them with immediate results. Or maybe it came from an innovative dieter who invented the plan while experimenting with foods he or she knew from experience could help take off pounds more quickly and easily than others.

In any event, we know that the Cabbage Soup Diet isn't new. Some Internet users remember a cabbage soup–based diet from fifteen years ago. A dietitian at Sacred Heart Medical Center in Eugene, Oregon, said this diet might be thirty years old or older!

That its origins are not known, and that it was almost certainly not developed by a major health institution, is a problem for some people. We tend to place our faith in the effectiveness of a diet developed by well-known experts. And, of course, those weight-loss plans created or endorsed by a major hospital, medical research organization, or well-known and well-placed obesity specialist have a certain cachet.

But not all experts are equal, and not all share similar views. Experts certainly have been known to question the merits of diets developed by other experts. Some of the high-protein, high-fat, low-carbohydrate diets that are the basis of several best-selling books are subjects of controversy, for example. Although these diets were developed by well-known weight-loss specialists, many doctors and nutrition experts have been highly critical of these plans. Even the famed Food Pyramid and Diet Guidelines, developed by experts at the United States Department of Agriculture, have come under attack recently, mainly because of what other, equally noted experts see as an overemphasis on carbohydrate foods.

So, while it may be reassuring to follow a diet planned by an expert, it is important to keep in mind that even experts disagree and that there is more to a good weight-loss plan than a noted author.

Whether it is a "mystery" diet or one created by a world-famous expert, a good weight-loss plan must meet certain criteria. If it's a diet you plan to follow for weeks or months, ask yourself: Is it well balanced? Does it supply adequate amounts of all the nutrients needed for good health. Or is it lopsided, requiring you to choose from one or two food categories and forbidding certain others? Just as important, can you imagine living with the diet for the duration?

When you use the Cabbage Soup Diet as it was meant to be used—for periods no longer than a week at a time, followed by two weeks of sensible eating—this unique food plan is safe, healthful, and gets results. It's packed with an abundance of vegetables and fruits and is very low in fat. As thousands of dieters know from experience, it's the best quick weight-loss plan around.

During the seven-day Cabbage Soup Diet cycle, you'll be supplying your body with all the nutrients it needs for good health. However, the diet does not supply all of them every day. That's one of the reasons you are urged to stop the diet for two weeks after you've finished a seven-day cycle and shift into a nutritionally well-balanced, moderate food plan, or the Cabbage Soup Maintenance Plan, for at least two weeks before repeating the diet.

As you will soon discover, the Cabbage Soup Diet will keep you feeling full and satisfied, so you can easily live with it, and on it, for the full seven-day cycle. As for its effectiveness, it will practically melt off the pounds, leaving you noticeably slimmer in just one week. At that point, your body and mind will be more prepared than ever before to continue the weight-loss process on a sound, sensible diet intended for long-term use or to maintain your new weight with the Cabbage Soup Maintenance Plan.

WHO CAN USE THE CABBAGE SOUP DIET?

The Cabbage Soup Diet should not be used by children or adolescents. It is not appropriate for diabetics or people with certain other medical conditions. (Talk with your doctor before starting this diet to make sure it is appropriate for you.)

But the Cabbage Soup Diet is a superior quick weight-loss plan for almost everyone else, including first-time dieters and the chronically disappointed who have tried everything without success, women and men who have been fit and thin most of their lives but who are beginning to develop a small, five- or ten-pound "problem," as well as those who have been overweight since childhood.

A ONE-SIZE-FITS-ALL PLAN

You might even call the Cabbage Soup Diet a one-size-fits-all plan. It's that flexible.

- Want to lose the last few pounds you haven't been able to shake with an ordinary diet? Use the New Cabbage Soup diet for three days and blitz them off.
- Want to take off the five or ten pounds that piled on as a result of overenthusiastic holiday eating? A single seven-day cycle of the diet should do the trick.
- What about the twenty or thirty pounds that accumulated who knows how or when, and which make you look and feel years older than you are? The Cabbage Soup Diet gives you a number of options: Use it for seven days to jump-start your weight loss and achieve immediate, visible results, then finish up with a longer, slower, more moderate regimen. *Or* use the Cabbage Soup Diet for a week, eat a normal, healthful diet for at least two weeks, and return for a second seven-day cycle of the diet. *Or* switch to the New Cabbage Soup Diet Maintenance Plan for two weeks and return to the Cabbage Soup Diet periodically.
- Got a major weight problem? Use the Cabbage Soup Diet for seven days to get motivated for long-term weight loss, then ask your doctor to suggest a safe,

well-balanced food plan to help you achieve a healthy weight.

A WORD TO THE WISE
Speak to your doctor before going on this or any other diet. Don't be surprised if he or she doesn't love the Cabbage Soup Diet, until you explain how you plan to use it: one week only, at intervals, or as a kickoff or wrap-up to another diet.

The Cabbage Soup Diet is strict, low in calories, and not meant to be a substitute for lifetime good nutrition. But the strictness and low calorie content are what make it such a miracle worker—and the one diet capable of solving common weight-loss problems other diets simply do not address.

FYI: A SNEAK PEEK AT THE PROTOTYPE
Now it's time to take a look at the original, unimproved Cabbage Soup Diet.

It was noted earlier in this chapter that there are several cabbage soup–based diets in circulation, including versions called the "Fat Burning Soup Diet," the "T-J Miracle Soup Diet," the "Rochester Diet," and the "Sacred Heart Hospital Diet." Each is a little different from the others, and it is likely that they evolved as individual dieters put their own personal spin on the basic plan. The version that follows, which came from the Internet, may be the prototype. Read through it, note the general principles, but don't use it. There's a new, improved, healthier version coming up in chapter 3.

THE BASIC CABBAGE SOUP DIET
You may have as much as you want of the mainstay of this diet—cabbage soup—and you can have it as often as you want throughout the day.

Note: Fruits and vegetables that are very low in calories are called "free" on the Cabbage Soup Diet. On certain days of the diet, you are allowed to have as many of these free fruits and vegetables as you want.

Day 1
Unlimited cabbage soup
Unlimited free fruits
Unsweetened tea or coffee if desired, cranberry juice, water

Day 2
Unlimited cabbage soup
Unlimited free vegetables
1 large baked potato with butter
Unsweetened tea or coffee if desired, cranberry juice, water

Day 3
Unlimited cabbage soup
Unlimited free fruit
Unlimited free vegetables
Unsweetened tea or coffee if desired, cranberry juice, water

Day 4
Unlimited cabbage soup
3 to 6 bananas
Skim milk, up to 8 glasses
Unsweetened tea or coffee if desired, cranberry juice, water

Day 5
Unlimited cabbage soup
10 to 20 ounces of lean beef or skinless chicken
1 28-ounce can of tomatoes or up to 6 fresh tomatoes
Unsweetened tea or coffee if desired, cranberry juice, water

Day 6
Unlimited cabbage soup
Unlimited lean beef

Unlimited free vegetables, including tomatoes
Unsweetened tea or coffee if desired, cranberry juice, water

Day 7
Unlimited cabbage soup
Unlimited brown rice
Unlimited free vegetables
Unsweetened tea or coffee if desired, cranberry juice, water

Remember, *do not* use this prototype diet. It's included here for reference only, to give you an idea of what the Cabbage Soup Diet is all about and to provide a basis of comparison to the New Cabbage Soup Diet coming up in chapter 3. The differences between the basic version and the new one may seem slight, yet they are significant. Nevertheless, the new version is right in line with the basic diet that thousands of people have used to achieve their personal weight goals.

MAGIC INGREDIENTS?

As you've seen, there are no strange or exotic foods on the Cabbage Soup Diet, only a wholesome and varied selection of the ordinary foods you've probably been eating all along.

There are a few unusual combinations, however, and some unexpected changes in content on Days 5 and 6. But "magic"? Hardly.

The origins of the diet may be a mystery, but there's no mystery about the healthful foods you'll be enjoying when you start your first seven-day cycle of Cabbage Soup Diet eating. There's no monumental weight-loss breakthrough here, either. Nothing but good foods that nutrition experts and ordinary dieters have known about for years.

In the next chapter we'll look more closely at the food, the plan, and the reasons why the Cabbage Soup Diet has become one of today's most talked about, most relied on, most effective quick weight-loss strategies.

CHAPTER 2

A Closer Look at the Cabbage Soup Diet

The original, or prototype, Cabbage Soup Diet in chapter 1 and the New Cabbage Soup Diet, to be revealed in chapter 3, have a lot of good things in common. They're equally effective at blitzing off pounds in a hurry. They're easy to follow and designed to help you feel comfortably full and satisfied from start to finish. Both versions of the diet offer almost instant results, so they help keep motivation high and provide the impetus needed to face down challenges and stay on track from the start of Day 1 to the end of Day 7 of the diet cycle. Many of the foods that make these diets—the basic, prototype version and the New Cabbage Soup Diet—such powerful, quick weight-loss tools are the same. And, of course, cabbage soup is the mainstay of both.

WHY SOUP?
For years, cabbage soup dieters have enjoyed the uniquely satisfying properties of a steaming bowl of great-tasting soup. They've experienced firsthand the way filling up on the soup blunts their appetite and makes weight loss easier. Science appears to back up their perceptions. A study by researchers at Pennsylvania State University, cited in the April 24, 1999, issue of *Science News* confirmed that filling

up on soup really does decrease appetite and increase weight loss.

This research confirmed that the body does not base its perceptions of "fullness" on the number of calories taken in but rather on the *volume* of food ingested. Further, it suggests that if water is added to food, increasing its volume, each calorie becomes more "filling." Hmmm. Food with water added. Sounds like soup, doesn't it?

The study was conducted in three parts on three separate days. Each day at lunchtime, twenty-four young women were given a 270-calorie appetizer portion of chicken and rice casserole. The casserole appetizer was served as is the first day. The second day, it was served along with a 10-ounce glass of water. On the third day, 10 ounces of water were mixed in with the chicken and rice, which was then served as soup. Each day, researchers measured how much lunch the women ate after finishing the casserole.

Results: On the days they ate the chicken and rice casserole and the chicken and rice plus glass of water, the women went on to consume an average of 300 calories for lunch. But on the days they had chicken and rice casserole diluted with water and served as soup, they took in an average of only 200 calories for lunch! The soup was that satisfying and that filling! And even though the women consumed fewer calories at lunchtime, they reported no increase in hunger in the afternoon. Nor did they eat more at dinner in the evening!

The researchers concluded that solid food and water affect hunger and feelings of fullness in different ways and that when water is processed as a food—as it is when we eat soup—it has a measurable effect on feelings of fullness and satisfaction after a meal.

It's proof of what cabbage soup dieters have known all along: There's nothing like soup to keep you feeling full and satisfied.

Of course, when the goal is to lose pounds, the ideal soup is healthful, nutritious, and low in calories.

DIET SOUP AND HEALTH SOUP

The miracle of cabbage soup is really that there is no miracle—aside from the fact that it is filling, satisfying, low in calories, and, like all good low-cal soups, makes losing weight faster and easier. It's also good tasting and wonderfully nutritious because it's made with a variety of vegetables rich in essential nutrients.

Cabbage is the "star" of this soup. It's quick-cooking, low in cost, and available in practically every supermarket throughout the year. Plus, it's packed with vitamins, making it a great nutritional bargain, particularly the humble, garden-variety cabbage you'll be using to make the soup. (White cabbage is traditional—and less expensive—but red can be used as well.)

Cabbage is high in fiber, vitamin C, and potassium. Its robust, earthy flavor is quickly suffused into the stock or broth it is cooked in. Cabbage is a member of the cruciferous family of vegetables (a few other crucifers are cauliflower, broccoli, and Brussels sprouts). Several studies suggest that women and men who consume large amounts of these vegetables are less likely to develop certain types of cancer, a benefit we'll be taking a closer look at later in this chapter. (Cancer-preventive vegetables, however, do *not* cure cancer.) Like many vegetables, cabbage is virtually fat-free. And it's so low in calories—a cup of raw shredded cabbage has only about 17—you could eat it by the pound and still lose weight. But, of course, you won't *need* to eat it by the pound on the Cabbage Soup Diet. You'll eat only as much as you want.

The other veggies in the basic soup recipe—carrots, red pepper, onions, green onions, and celery—are great nutritional bargains, too.

Carrots, like cabbage, provide fiber and are a rich source of cancer-protective beta-carotene, a provitamin A carotenoid. In fact, carrots are among the best ways to get beta-carotene into your diet: a ½-cup serving of cooked carrots provides more beta-carotene than you'd get in a similar portion of almost any other vegetable. At about 30 calories

---

Nutrition Update: Boning Up on Vegetables

Here's one more reason for upping your veggie intake on the Cabbage Soup Diet and for the rest of your life: In looking at the relationship between diet and bone health, scientists at the University of Aberdeen in Scotland found that a high intake of nutrients found in certain fruits and vegetables—especially fiber, vitamin C, potassium, and magnesium—appears to slow the development of osteoporosis in women. Among other factors important to strong bones are vitamin D, sunshine, and exercise.

---

per medium carrot, this vegetable offers an abundance of important nutrients at a very low cost in calories.

Green and red peppers provide vitamin C, are good sources of vitamin A carotenoids and potassium, and are very low in calories; 1 cup cubed green or red pepper has about 25 calories.

Onions, which contain potassium and some protein and fiber, add delectable flavor and aroma to the soup. A cup of cooked onion sliced into bite-size pieces has about 60 calories. Green onions, also part of the basic soup recipe, are better known as scallions in some parts of the country. They are long and stalklike in shape, with a small, rounded white "head" and edible green leaves. Green onions contribute a fair amount of potassium and fiber as well as traces of protein. Like bulb-shape onions, they enhance the flavor of the soup, and at a caloric cost of only about 35 calories per cup.

Tomatoes deliver good amounts of vitamins A and C and potassium, along with some niacin (a component of the B-vitamin complex), and are a good source of a possibly cancer-protective substance called lycopene. Their flavor adds richness and complexity to the soup. Tomatoes are composed mainly of water, so they are very low in calories; a whole pound of tomatoes contains only about 95! However, because they are condensed during the canning process, a cup of canned stewed tomatoes has about 90 calories.

Celery, the final vegetable in the basic soup recipe, contributes subtle flavor, fiber, and potassium to the mix. Like tomatoes, celery is mainly water, which accounts for its very low calorie content; a ½ cup of diced celery contains about 25 calories.

As you will see when you read through the new and improved version of the soup recipe in chapter 4, it contains all the healthful veggies listed above, plus another ingredient that makes it even more nutritious. However, the new version omits the high-sodium onion soup mix and bouillon called for in the original recipe. Omitting these high-sodium ingredients makes the soup a better food for those who must watch their salt intake. If you crave a saltier flavor and there's no particular reason for you to restrict your sodium intake, you can always add salt at the table.

THE SOUP WITH "PHYTE"

Packed with vitamins and low in fat and calories, Cabbage Soup Diet vegetables are rich in health-protective phytochemicals (pronounced fight-o-chemicals). These are nutrients that the International Food Information Council describes as containing "significant levels of biologically active components that impart health benefits beyond basic nutrition when consumed in typical or optimal serving sizes."

Research suggests that many of these biologically active substances may reduce the risk of a range of killer diseases, including the ones responsible for more than 60 percent of all deaths annually in the United States—among them many cancers, heart disease, and stroke. The potential benefits of phytochemicals don't stop there, however; they also appear to be protective against cataracts, osteoporosis, and even urinary tract infections!

Phytochemicals aren't new, of course. They've always been present in the ordinary fruits, vegetables, grains, and other plant foods that have been part of the human diet for thousands of years. But it wasn't until recently that scientists began to explore their role in keeping us healthy. Now phytochemicals are the subject of some of today's hottest nutrition news—and we haven't heard the last word yet. Investigators have discovered more than nine hundred different phytochemicals in plant foods and expect to identify many more as research into this exciting new field continues.

The cabbage soup you'll be enjoying on the diet—as well as many of the other foods you will eat during each seven-day cycle—is rich in health-promoting phytochemicals. Let's look at just a few.

ANTIOXIDANTS

As we've seen, some of the vegetables included in the basic cabbage soup recipe are good sources of vitamin C and beta-carotene, both of which are phytochemicals with antioxidant properties that are important to our health and well-being.

How do antioxidants work? To simplify, as our bodies use oxygen to create energy, groups of atoms called "free radicals" are produced. These by-products can damage cells throughout our bodies and interfere with the DNA that controls cell growth. Large numbers of damaged cells make us more vulnerable to many diseases, including some cancers, heart disease, stroke, and cataracts. Free radical formation is natural, inevitable, and can't be prevented. But some of the damage caused by free radicals can be lessened by antioxidant substances in the foods we eat. These substances surround and neutralize free radicals, rendering them less harmful. So when we consume foods that deliver ample amounts of antioxidants, we're actually helping to keep our cells intact and healthier, reducing our risk for many diseases, and slowing the degeneration that takes place in our bodies over the years.

Among the "big gun" antioxidants in food are vitamin C, beta-carotene, vitamin E, and selenium.

Vitamin C, also called ascorbic acid, is a water-soluble vitamin found in all body fluids, so it may be one of our first lines of defense. The body does not store this powerful antioxidant, so it's important to get some vitamin C daily. That's exactly what you will be doing on the Cabbage Soup Diet, since vitamin C is plentiful in cabbage and green peppers as well as in broccoli, green leafy vegetables, and many of the other free fruits and vegetables you will be filling up on during each seven-day cycle.

Beta-carotene protects dark green, yellow, and orange vegetables and fruits from solar radiation damage; in humans, it may reduce cancer risk and helps maintain a healthy immune system. Tomatoes and carrots, important ingredients in the cabbage soup that is the basis of this diet, are good sources of beta-carotene. Other good sources are squash, broccoli, sweet potatoes, kale, collard greens, cantaloupe, peaches, and apricots.

Vitamin E, a fat-soluble vitamin, may help prevent or delay coronary heart disease and appears to interfere with the formation of nitrosamines, which are carcinogens formed in the stomach when certain foods are consumed. Vitamin E also contributes to a healthy immune system. Good sources are wheat germ; vegetable oils; tofu; canned apricots and peaches; nectarines; greens such as dandelion greens, kohlrabi, turnip greens, and mustard greens; broccoli; sprouts; spinach; eggs; chicken; turkey; liver; clams; fish such as mackerel, ocean perch, and salmon; scallops; shrimp; multigrain and fortified cereals; peanut butter, peanuts, and other nuts, including Brazil nuts, almonds, and filberts. Some of these foods have a place in the Cabbage Soup Diet, but many other foods rich in vitamin E do not, so you may want to talk to your doctor about taking a multivitamin and mineral supplement while you are on the diet.

Selenium is an essential trace mineral with antioxidant properties. Some studies indicate that the risk of heart disease, as well as the death rate from lung, colorectal, and prostate cancers, is lower among people who consume good amounts of selenium-rich foods. Selenium is present in many veggies, including the ones you will use to prepare the cabbage soup. However, the amount of selenium in food is directly related to the amount of selenium in the soil it was grown in, so once again, if you are concerned about getting adequate amounts of this mineral, on this diet or otherwise, check with your doctor about taking a multivitamin and mineral supplement that includes selenium. Good sources of selenium are kidney, liver, wheat germ, wheat bran, tuna, mackerel, onions, tomatoes, broccoli, eggs, chicken, and garlic.

Warning: **Do not overdose with nutritional supplements containing more than the Recommended Daily Allowance (RDA) of these or other nutrients.** Some vitamins, minerals, and other nutrients—including but not limited to beta-carotene and selenium—are toxic when taken in large amounts. The best way to get adequate amounts of essential nutrients is through a balanced diet that supplies a variety of foods. However, in some circumstances— such as when you are following a reduced-calorie diet like this one—a good multivitamin and mineral supplement may be advisable. When in doubt, get advice from your doctor.

Tip: Some of the most beneficial phytochemicals are pigments—compounds that give plants their color. Bright yellow, orange, red, green, and purple fruits and vegetables tend to be especially rich in phytochemicals and other nutrients.

Here's a rundown of some of the other health-promoting phytochemicals you will be consuming on the Cabbage Soup Diet:

Ajoene   A naturally occurring compound found in garlic, ajoene may reduce the risk of stroke and heart disease. Because the more we learn about it, the more impressive this aromatic vegetable becomes, we've added garlic to the new, improved cabbage soup recipe.

Allyl Sulfides   Onions, garlic, leeks, chives, and shallots all have good amounts of allyl sulfides, compounds that may inhibit cancer by neutralizing cancer-causing chemicals in the body. These compounds also are thought to help lower blood cholesterol and blood pressure and may protect against heart disease.

Butyl Phthalide   This compound is what gives celery its distinctive flavor and aroma. Butyl phthalide is thought to help protect against high blood pressure and high cholesterol levels. You'll be getting plenty of it in the soup.

Indoles   Found throughout nature, these aromatic compounds assist the body in ridding itself of toxins through excretion. Some researchers believe the indoles in cabbage, broccoli, Brussels sprouts, and their related plants are what give these vegetables their cancer-preventive properties.

Lycopene   The compound that gives tomatoes and many other red vegetables their brilliant color, lycopene may protect against certain cancers, including cancers of the stomach, bladder, cervix, and colon. A Harvard University study found that men who ate several servings a week of tomatoes and tomato-based products lowered their risk for prostate cancer by half. (Surprise: The lycopene in cooked tomatoes is more easily absorbed than that in fresh raw tomatoes!) Red peppers, another ingredient in the cabbage soup, also contains good amounts of lycopene.

Coumarin   Also found in tomatoes, coumarin may help prevent blood clots.

The vitamins, minerals, and phytochemicals present in the cabbage soup vegetables and other elements of the diet are important for optimal health. But they're not the only valuable components of the Cabbage Soup Diet. Fiber deserves a few brief paragraphs, too.

THE FIBER FACTOR

Dietary fiber is found in the nondigestible parts of fruits and vegetables—the seeds, the skin, the hulls of unrefined grains—and supplies bulk to the diet. Fiber has practically no nutritive value, and, unlike vitamins, it is not essential to human life and growth. Yet it is very important to good nutrition and plays an important role in both the old and the new versions of the Cabbage Soup Diet. Fiber, you see, appears to increase the amount of fat excreted by the body, which in turn may accelerate weight loss. Fiber certainly fills you up at little or no cost in calories, as scientific research has borne out. In one study, volunteers who were served a diet high in fiber consumed significantly fewer calories than they did normally, even though they were instructed to eat as much as they wanted.

Whether your goal is to lose weight or maintain it, there are many good reasons to get plenty of fiber into your diet.

- *Fiber is absorbent.* Because it soaks up water and begins to swell as it passes through the upper part of the digestive tract, fiber promotes long-lasting feelings of fullness.
- *Fiber itself is nonnutritive and delivers no calories, so it fills you up with without adding to your calorie intake for the day.* (Of course, not all high-fiber foods are low in calories—especially if you doctor them up with fatty add-ons like butter or oil.)
- *High-fiber foods require lots of chewing.* This extra chewing slows down your rate of eating and allows time for satiety signals to reach your brain before you go overboard.
- *Fiber, because it is so filling, also tends to reduce your calorie intake by "displacing" other, higher-*

calorie foods. After a high-fiber first course, you just won't be as eager for the food that follows.

• *Fiber also helps keep blood sugar levels steadier by slowing the digestion of carbohydrates.* Low blood sugar can make you feel fatigued or irritable, and when blood sugar levels swing down low enough, your body will respond by calling out for more food.

As you probably know already, there are many other advantages to be gained by consuming good amounts of fiber. There is evidence, for instance, that certain types of fiber reduce the amount of fat and cholesterol in the bloodstream; this in turn may decrease the risk of heart disease. A high-fiber diet also appears to lower colon cancer risk and makes appendicitis and diverticulosis (a disease in which the walls of the intestines develop small "pockets") less likely. Fiber research is ongoing. This important substance in our food may turn out to have many more health benefits than the ones we already know about.

Actually, there are two kinds of fiber, soluble and insoluble. The soluble kind forms a gel when mixed with liquid during digestion. It helps lower blood cholesterol and keeps blood sugar levels on an even keel. Insoluble fiber passes through the digestive tract as is and is associated with a reduced risk of colon cancer, diverticulosis, and appendicitis. The vegetables that go into the cabbage soup mainstay of this diet deliver both types of fiber in abundance.

Cabbage soup is indeed health soup, packed with vital nutrients, and it's great eating on a diet or off. But when weight loss is the goal, what's equally important about the original cabbage soup recipe and the new, improved version is that they also are low in calories and fat.

CALORIES DO COUNT

Many of the vegetable ingredients of the soup as well as the "free" vegetables you'll be consuming on the diet are so low in calories that you can eat huge amounts of them without taking in the minimum number of calories you need each day to maintain your weight. Some of these vegetables actually provide fewer calories than your body expends in chewing, swallowing, and digesting them. The negative calorie value of these vegetables helps explain why you can fill up on the soup four or five times a day—or more—if you want to, never feel hungry, and still experience dramatic weight loss in seven days.

Overall, on the Cabbage Soup Diet you are going to be eating fewer calories than you're used to. Perhaps the idea of denying your body the calories it needs may make you a little uncomfortable. But there are only two ways to lose pounds. One is to consume fewer, more healthful calories; the other is to burn off greater numbers of calories through exercise. It would be difficult to find a doctor or nutrition expert who did not encourage you to do both. And later in this book you will find tips and suggestions for healthy lifetime eating, including the New Cabbage Soup Diet Maintenance Plan, plus ideas for tailoring a fitness plan you'll be able to live with—and enjoy—for the rest of your life.

But the New Cabbage Soup Diet was created to blast off up to ten pounds in seven days. It's not meant to be used for extended periods. Low-calorie and negative-calorie foods are part of what make it so effective. If you are healthy and do not have a chronic medical condition such as diabetes, the New Cabbage Soup Diet is a safe, sure way to solve a minor weight problem, shape up for a big event, kick-off a long-term diet, and/or shake off the last few pounds after months on a slow weight-loss plan.

The very-low-calorie and negative-calorie aspects of the New Cabbage Soup Diet make it a distant relative of some of the low-calorie diets you remember from the past. These weight-loss plans typically restricted the dieter to a very limited selection of low-calories foods, such as grapefruit, or rice, or salad greens, and they usually stressed consuming no more than a certain number of calories each day. The New Cabbage Soup Diet is different; while you are on it, you will be eating a wide variety of foods, but not all of them every day. And, of course, you'll never have to count a single calorie!

THE FETISH FOR LOW FAT

The New Cabbage Soup Diet and the old are both low in calories and low in fat, which is the most concentrated source of calories. But except for plain, no-fat yogurt and fat-reduced salad dressing, which are part of the new version of the diet, you won't be using commercially produced low-fat versions of ordinary foods. No low-fat cookies or cake. No low-fat snack foods. No low-fat frozen desserts.

The rise in popularity of reduced-fat products and the anti-fat fetish of the last decade or so may have contributed to what some health officials have called the "obesity epidemic" of recent years. Those experts are referring to the increase in the percentage of overweight Americans in the 1980s and 1990s, as documented by a long-term study conducted by the federal Centers for Disease Control and Prevention, and by the 1999 National Health and Nutrition Examination Survey, which found that 34 percent of U.S. adults aged 20 to 74 years are overweight and an additional 27 percent are obese. The following chart says it all.

Increase in Prevalence (%) of Overweight (BMI ≥ 25), Obesity (BMI ≥ 30), and Severe Obesity (BMI ≥ 40) among U.S. Adults			
	Overweight (BMI ≥ 25)	Obesity (BMI ≥ 30)	Severe Obesity (BMI ≥ 40)
1999–2000	64.5	30.5	4.7
1988–1994	56.0	23.0	2.9
1976–1980	46.0	14.4	No data

Sources: Centers for Disease Control, National Center for Health Statistics, *National Health and Nutritional Examination Survey: United States, 2002*; Katherine M. Flegal et al., "Prevalance and Trends in Obesity among U.S. Adults, 1999–2000," *Journal of the American Medical Association* 288 (2002): 1723–27; National Institutes of Health, National Heart, Lung, and Blood Institute, and National Institute of Diabetes and Digestive and Kidney Disease, *Clinical Guidelines on the Identification, Evaluation, and Treatment of Overweight and Obesity in Adults* (Washington, D.C.: 1998).

The percentage increase seems to have little to do with the aging of the population because it is evident in all age groups. For example, today's forty-year-olds on average weigh more than forty-year-olds did in the 1970s. It's the same with children, young adults, and older people.

What has happened since the mid-1970s? For one thing, a barrage of reports and studies began to appear linking a high-fat diet to heart disease, various types of cancer, diabetes, and other conditions—including, of course, obesity. Soon a spate of magazine articles and best-selling books citing dietary fat as the primary and even the sole factor in obesity were published. At the same time, food technologists were developing methods of producing a wide range of products using less fat, and these items began to show up in supermarkets with phrases like "lower fat," "reduced fat," or "fat-free" on their labels. Millions of Americans, newly aware of the importance of consuming less fat, began to use them.

Unfortunately, too often people interpreted the words "low fat" on a food label to mean "go ahead, eat all you want." And we did. The logic went something like this: Fat was the designated culprit. Fat makes you fat, and fat makes you more vulnerable to killer diseases. So far so good. But then we made the leap from there to the false notion that we could load up with foods that were no fat, low fat, or fat reduced without gaining weight. Few of us understood or took into consideration that in many of these products, sweeteners and other high-calorie carbohydrate ingredients were used to replace some of the flavor that was lost when the fat was removed.

Low fat isn't the same as low calorie. And in fact, many reduced-fat foods, such as lower-fat ice creams, are laden with calories; some are even higher in calories than their higher-fat counterparts! So when Americans started filling up on low-fat but calorific foods, the gross national weight began to skyrocket and the obesity epidemic was under way. This scenario is only one put forward by public health experts to explain why millions of Americans weigh more now than their counterparts did in the 1970s, but it is an important one.

Today reputable health and diet experts are no longer urging Americans to purge as much fat from their diets as possible—nor are they recommending a return to the old days of high-fat eating. Rather, instead of focusing on reducing total fat intake, they are encouraging us to consume fats in moderation and to replace "bad" fats (the saturated kind) with "good" fats (polyunsaturated and monounsaturated). The New Cabbage Soup Maintenance Plan (introduced in chapter 19), which includes moderate amounts of "good" fats, was designed with this new thinking in mind.

While you are on the Cabbage Soup Diet, however, both your calorie intake and fat consumption will be low enough to force your body to give up as many pounds as possible in each seven-day cycle.

As we've seen in this up-close look at what makes the Cabbage Soup Diet work, the food you'll be eating on this unique weight-loss plan is much more than just good diet food. It's good, healthful food, good for anyone, anytime. In the next chapter, you'll find out why the New Cabbage Soup Diet is even better than the old one.

CHAPTER 3

The New and Improved Cabbage Soup Diet Revealed

Why on earth change the Cabbage Soup Diet? It's already one of the most popular, most talked and written about, most successful quick weight-loss programs ever. It already has dieters from coast to coast (and on the other side of the Atlantic, too) raving about the dramatic results they've seen in seven days or less. It's already the most highly effective and versatile approach to a range of problems:

- You can use it for three days anytime you need to slim down enough to fit into a favorite dress or suit for a big event.
- You can follow the seven-day version for a visible, ten-pound loss that makes a major difference in the way you look and feel.
- You can use the diet as a quick-start, highly motivational kick-off to a slower, long-term weight-loss program that will leave you not only slimmer but also healthier and less vulnerable to serious diseases.
- And you can use it repeatedly—up to three times in a three-month period—as long as you allow at least two weeks between each diet cycle.

So why change the diet? For two simple reasons. To make sure you get even better, quicker results. And to make it more nutritious.

Even though the original, unmodified Cabbage Soup Diet gives you the solution to just about any diet problem, there was room for improvement. The New Cabbage Soup Diet is equally good for addressing those problems, plus it's better for you and even easier to follow.

WHAT'S WRONG WITH THE ORIGINAL CABBAGE SOUP DIET?

The original Cabbage Soup Diet calls for an abundance of good, healthful food. But if you review the original, proto-type diet in chapter 1, you will see that some important food groups are excluded or almost absent and one type of food is overused. The old version is deficient in the following areas:

Protein In recent decades, the need for protein, especially animal protein, has been revised downward. Nevertheless, it is important to consume some protein on a daily basis, whether you are on a diet or not. The original Cabbage Soup Diet supplied very little protein except on Days 5 and 6, when unlimited amounts of beef or chicken were allowed.

Grains There are no grains on the old Cabbage Soup Diet other than the brown rice on Day 7. Grains are important sources of fiber, and whole grains provide important B vitamins and some iron at a relatively low cost in calories.

Calcium The old version of the diet is too low in calcium except on Day 4, when you are instructed to drink eight glasses of skim milk. Calcium, of course, is essential for maintaining strong bones and teeth and to help prevent bone loss in adults. Osteoporosis, a condition in which bones become porous and fragile, is a major health problem in many older people. Adequate calcium throughout life can help reduce the risk for this disease in later years.

Beef The original Cabbage Soup Diet allows large amounts of beef on Days 5 and 6. Although there is a place for moderate amounts of red meat on any sensible, long-term food plan, beef is a source of saturated fats and cholesterol and is too high in calories for optimal, quick weight loss.

The Boredom Factor   The original Cabbage Soup Diet is long on plain, wholesome food but short on variety. The original Cabbage Soup Diet provided nothing in the way of flavor variations, and the result is a certain bland sameness from meal to meal and day to day. Variety is important. It's a source of gratification and satisfaction in itself. And think about this: Interesting food, because it helps us feel less deprived, can help us stay committed to the weight-loss process.

MUCH BETTER—THE NEW CABBAGE SOUP DIET
The New Cabbage Soup Diet, which offers better nutrition, more variety—and better results—addresses all of the just-mentioned shortcomings of the old Cabbage Soup Diet.

PROTEIN BOOST!
Your muscles, organs, glands—in short, your whole body— are constructed of proteins and require protein for growth, development, and maintenance.

"Animal" Protein   As you probably remember from high school or college nutrition or health courses, proteins are made up of twenty or so amino acids, nine of which are not produced in the human body. Foods of animal origin, such as meat and fish, eggs, milk, cheese and other dairy products, as well as some soybean-based foods, deliver complete protein, the kind that provides the nine essential amino acids.

The protein content of the New Cabbage Soup Diet gets a boost with the inclusion of your choice of plain, no-fat yogurt or skim milk, both foods of animal origin that provide essential amino acids. On the new version of the diet, you will be enjoying eight ounces of either of these foods every day.

Note: Switching between skim milk and plain, no-fat yogurt in the course of a single day is not allowed. You must decide at the beginning of each day if it's to be a milk day or a yogurt day.

"Plant" Protein   Many plant foods also supply significant amounts of protein, but with the exception of soybeans, no single plant—grain, vegetable, or fruit—supplies *all* the essential amino acids. For that reason, protein from plants is sometimes referred to as "incomplete."

However, when your diet includes a variety of plant foods, chances are good that you will be getting adequate amounts of complete protein. That's because different plant foods supply different combinations of amino acids. If you consume a variety of vegetables and other foods of plant origin, as you will be doing on the New Cabbage Soup Diet, the various amino acids combined will produce the complete proteins your body needs.

To give you a wider variety of plant foods from which your body can pick and choose to make complete proteins, brown rice has been added to each day of the New Cabbage Soup Diet. You will be consuming it as an ingredient in the cabbage soup in amounts that provide you with approximately ¼ cup brown rice each day. (The exact amount will depend on how much soup you consume.)

Debunking a Protein Myth

One of the older "musts" of good nutrition has been proven wrong. Nutrition scientists used to believe that the only way to make sure the body got complete protein from plant foods was to eat a grain product (such as rice, bread, or pasta), with beans, peas, or lentils at the same meal. Now they recognize that combining these food elements at a single sitting isn't necessary. Eating a variety of plant foods over the course of a day or so can be enough.

RICE IS NICE

The same brown rice that boosts the protein content of the soup also makes up for some of the diet's grain deficiency. Brown rice is specified because it is richer in vitamins, fiber, and other nutrients than white rice.

To understand the difference, first imagine a grain of rice in its natural state. It's covered with a tough husk. Under that there's a layer of bran. The bran layer surrounds the endosperm. In polished white rice, the husk and bran are removed, leaving only the endosperm and germ. Brown rice, however, retains most of the bran. Bran is what gives brown rice its darker color, nuttier flavor, chewier texture, and more and better nutrients—including larger amounts of quality plant protein, more fiber, more B-complex vitamins, some vitamin E, and potassium. Nutritionally, brown rice wins out over white hands down. The only drawback: Brown rice takes somewhat longer to prepare. Never mind. Fifteen minutes more in cooking time is a small price to pay for the increase in important nutritional elements you get in return.

CALCIUM UPGRADE

Rice does double duty on the New Cabbage Soup Diet by contributing vegetable protein and supplying fiber as well as good amounts of the important nutrients found in grains. The skim milk or yogurt you will be eating every day on the new version of the diet is also a two-for-one addition. As we have seen, both provide more complete protein—and both contribute calcium to the diet.

Nutritional studies suggest that three out of four adults, whether they are dieting or not, do not get enough calcium. That's not good, because calcium is crucial to maintaining strong bones. Consuming milk and milk products, such as yogurt, is one of the best ways to supply your body with calcium, which is why the New Cabbage Soup Diet includes 1 cup skim milk or plain low-fat or no-fat yogurt daily. (Removing the fat from these foods does not reduce their calcium content. Skim milk and no-fat yogurt deliver as much calcium as do equal amounts of whole milk or regular yogurt.)

To be sure, 1 cup of either of these two foods does not supply your body's total daily requirement of this important mineral. Dietitians typically recommend a minimum of 2 cups milk or yogurt daily, plus several servings of other calcium-rich foods, to ensure adequate calcium intake. To augment the calcium you get from milk or yogurt, choose vegetables with a high calcium content on days when unlimited free vegetables are on the New Cabbage Soup Diet menu.

Good Vegetable Sources of Calcium

Have at least one of these low-calorie vegetable sources of calcium on days when free vegetables are part of the diet.

Leafy green vegetables: romaine lettuce, spinach, escarole, collard greens, kale, watercress, chicory, and parsley

Nonleafy vegetables: broccoli, cauliflower, asparagus

Nutrition Extra: To further bone up on calcium, ask your doctor about taking a multivitamin and mineral supplement.

WHERE'S THE BEEF?

As we've seen, the original Cabbage Soup Diet allows you to have up to 20 ounces of beef on Day 5 and as much beef as you like on Day 6. That's too much beef. All types of beef, including hamburger, contain fat and cholesterol. Even if the beef is lean to begin with, and even if you trim away as much visible fat as you can, it's impossible to avoid fat and cholesterol entirely when you eat beef.

Better protein choices that are lower in fat, cholesterol,

and calories are grilled, roasted, or broiled chicken or grilled or broiled fish. Do these replacements really make a big difference? The answer is a resounding "Yes!"

There are about 197 calories in 4 ounces of very lean broiled ground beef and about 242 calories in 4 ounces of broiled lean T-bone steak. But there are only 159 calories in 4 ounces of broiled halibut and 149 calories in broiled snapper. As for chicken, one broiled chicken breast without the skin has 108 calories, and one drumstick without skin has 76 calories.

To keep calories, fat, and cholesterol in the diet as low as possible and yet provide good amounts of complete protein, the New Cabbage Soup Diet omits beef and instead calls for unlimited grilled, broiled, or roasted fish or chicken on Days 5 and 6. Your choice! And you are free to alternate between fish or chicken at lunch and dinner on both days.

GOOD-FOR-YOU-GARLIC

Over the centuries, garlic (sometimes referred to as the "stinking rose") has been the bane of fictional vampires as well as a popular folk remedy in many cultures. Now modern researches are taking a second look at this pungent bulb and finding that it may indeed have health-protective properties. The phytochemical ajoene was mentioned in chapter 2. This chemical, part of the compound that gives garlic its characteristic aroma and flavor, is a proven anticoagulant (blood thinner) and is thought to help reduce the risk of stroke and heart disease. Ajoene also has antimicrobial properties, which inhibit the growth of both bacteria and fungi.

On the New Cabbage Soup Diet, you will be helping yourself to the benefits of garlic every time you enjoy the soup, because garlic is now part of the basic soup recipe. Don't like the smell or taste of garlic? Not to worry. You will be using only small amounts—small enough that you'll hardly know it's there!

PUMPED-UP FLAVOR

The old Cabbage Soup Diet didn't mention any flavoring ingredients, not even salt and pepper. Since we don't know who created the diet, it's impossible to ask if there was a reason for this omission or whether it was just an oversight.

What we do know, however, is that there are dozens of no-fat, no-cal, and very-low-cal ways to add more zing to the diet. So, because taste appeal is important even on a quick weight-loss plan such as this one, a range of seasonings and other flavor ingredients has been added.

On the New Cabbage Soup Diet, you can perk up your food with your choice of fresh or dried herbs, spices, hot sauces, soy sauce, vinegars, or lemon juice—in short, with just about any no-cal or low-cal flavoring ingredients you can think of. You can also use 1 tablespoon per day of your favorite no- or low-calorie prepared salad dressings.

Oils and oil-based salad dressings, rich sauces, butter, margarine, and other high-fat or high-calorie condiments are taboo, of course.

In chapter 9, you will find suggestions and ideas for pumping up the flavor of all the foods on the New Cabbage Soup Diet, including the soup.

OTHER NEW CABBAGE SOUP DIET CHANGES IN BRIEF

The Major Change on Day 7

If you look at the old Cabbage Soup Diet plan in chapter 1, you will see that on Day 7 you are directed to eat as much cabbage soup as you want and also to have unlimited amounts of brown rice, unlimited amounts of free vegetables, and as much unsweetened fruit juice as you care to drink. The cabbage soup, of course, is part of every day on the diet. It's not clear why the person who originated this unique weight-loss plan decided that people should fill up on brown rice that day, or what purpose is served by drinking all that fruit juice. The directive to fill up on brown rice and fruit juice on Day 7 seems pointless and arbitrary, in fact.

As you know, many who have used the Cabbage Soup Diet were thrilled with the quick weight loss they achieved, and there are times when it's best not to quarrel with success. However, this isn't one of them.

Since brown rice is now an ingredient in the new cabbage soup recipe and you will be receiving some of its nutritional advantages every day, there's no longer any need for unlimited brown rice on Day 7.

As for all the unsweetened fruit juice, juice does deliver most of the nutrients you would get in whole fruit. But it's not as filling and satisfying, and it provides less fiber. The question is, why unlimited fruit juice on Day 7 instead of unlimited fruit? Although the juice may offer a nice change of pace for people who prefer it to whole, fresh fruit, there is no logical answer to the question. Therefore, the unlimited fruit juice on Day 7 has been removed.

Day 7 of the New Cabbage Soup Diet now offers unlimited soup, unlimited vegetables, and unlimited fruit. It is, in fact, identical to Day 4 and a much more satisfying and logical way to end the seven-day diet cycle.

No Cranberry Juice
The reason for excluding cranberry juice as a drink option in the new version of the diet is simple. There are approximately 144 calories in a cup of cranberry juice cocktail, and although it tastes good and contributes vitamin C to the diet, the cost in calories just isn't worth it.

Olive Oil Instead of Butter
Many dieters are surprised, when they glance through the meal plans that made up the original version of the diet, to see butter included as an accompaniment to baked potato on Day 3. A healthier option is to drizzle olive oil on your baked potato.

What? Olive oil on a baked potato? Yes, indeed. Butter, a saturated fat, has about 102 calories and 31 milligrams of cholesterol per tablespoon. A tablespoon of olive oil has about the same number of calories but no cholesterol. Plus, it's high in monounsaturated fatty acids, which help lower blood levels of LDL cholesterol. (LDL cholesterol—sometimes referred to as "bad" cholesterol—is the kind that can build up in the arteries, forming the artery-clogging plaque that puts us at greater risk for heart attack or stroke.) Those same fatty acids in olive oil also protect HDL cholesterol (the "good" cholesterol), which some scientists believe works against the development of plaque.

As for taste, olive oil has a luscious, almost nutlike flavor you're sure to savor once you try it on your potato. You may even discover you prefer it to butter!

> **Tip:** Extra virgin olive oil is the most expensive, the most flavorful, and the favorite of olive oil connoisseurs. However, if you are cautious by nature, start with a milder olive oil. These sometimes have the word "light" or "mild" on the label.

Artificial Sweetener for Tea and Coffee

You are allowed your choice of tea, coffee and/or water at every meal while you're on the New Cabbage Soup Diet. The old version of the diet specified unsweetened tea or coffee. It's not hard to understand why sugar, at 23 calories a packet, was prohibited. But there's no reason why you shouldn't use an artificial sweetener at 4 calories a packet. So, if you want to sweeten your favorite beverage with an artificial sweetener, go ahead! As for diet soda, it's a no-no. Gas is a concern for some people following the New Cabbage Soup Diet, so carbonated (gassy) drinks should be avoided.

There you have it, the changes that make the New Cabbage Soup Diet healthier and better tasting than the original— but just as effective for crashing off pounds in a hurry.

Read on for the details of your actual eating plan.

THE NEW CABBAGE SOUP DIET

Now here's how the New Cabbage Soup Diet stacks up. Rest assured, the new version is right in line with the basic diet that thousands of people have used to achieve their personal weight goals—only healthier and easier to stick with!

Day 1

> Unlimited cabbage soup
> Unlimited free fruits
> 1 tablespoon low- or no-fat salad dressing
> Your choice of herbs, spices, or other flavoring
> > ingredients
> 1 8-ounce serving of skim milk or plain, low-fat or
> > no-fat yogurt
> Tea or coffee if desired, plain or with artificial
> > sweetener
> Water

Day 2

> Unlimited cabbage soup
> Unlimited free vegetables
> 1 large baked potato, plain or with olive oil
> Your choice of herbs, spices, or other flavoring
> > ingredients
> 1 8-ounce serving of skim milk or plain, low-fat or
> > no-fat yogurt
> Tea or coffee if desired, plain or with artificial
> > sweetener
> Water

Day 3

> Unlimited cabbage soup
> Unlimited free vegetables
> Unlimited free fruits
> Your choice of herbs, spices, or other flavoring
> > ingredients

1 8-ounce serving of skim milk or plain, low-fat or
     no-fat yogurt
Tea or coffee if desired, plain or with artificial
     sweetener
Water

Day 4

Unlimited cabbage soup
3 to 6 bananas
Your choice of herbs, spices, or other flavoring
     ingredients
1 8-ounce serving of skim milk or plain, low-fat or
     no-fat yogurt
Tea or coffee if desired, plain or with artificial
     sweetener
Water

Day 5

Unlimited cabbage soup
Unlimited broiled or grilled fish
Unlimited broiled or grilled chicken
1 28-ounce can tomatoes or up to 6 fresh tomatoes
Your choice of herbs, spices, or other flavoring
     ingredients
1 8-ounce serving of skim milk or plain, low-fat or
     no-fat yogurt
Tea or coffee if desired, plain or with artificial
     sweetener
Water

Day 6

Unlimited cabbage soup
Unlimited broiled or grilled fish
Unlimited broiled or grilled chicken
Unlimited free vegetables, including tomatoes
Your choice of herbs, spices, or other flavoring
     ingredients

1 8-ounce serving of skim milk or plain, low-fat or
    no-fat yogurt
Tea or coffee if desired, plain or with artificial
    sweetener
Water

Day 7

Unlimited cabbage soup
Unlimited free fruits
Your choice of herbs, spices, or other flavoring
    ingredients
1 8-ounce serving of skim milk or plain, low-fat or
    no-fat yogurt
Tea or coffee if desired, plain or with artificial
    sweetener
Water

There you have it. Brown rice and garlic in the soup, skim milk or yogurt every day, artificial sweetener, 1 tablespoon low- or no-fat salad dressing, healthful olive oil on your potato, your choice of no-cal seasonings—no beef, no butter, and no cranberry juice. Those are the simple changes that make the New Cabbage Soup Diet tastier, healthier, and even better for getting rid of pounds in a hurry.

In the next chapter, you'll learn how to prepare the soup and find out even more about the nutritious foods you'll be enjoying when you start your first cycle of the New Cabbage Soup Diet, including the best free fruits and vegetables and how to shop for them and what kinds of fish and chicken are lowest in fat.

CHAPTER 4

Super Soup—How to Make It

Now you know about the healthful foods that make up the New Cabbage Soup Diet, and you know which foods to eat on each of the seven days in the diet cycle. You're almost ready for your first week of the diet and the speedy results you'll get with it.

But this amazing diet, like every other weight-loss plan you've ever tried or heard about, requires some advance planning. Most important, you'll need to make the soup.

NOT A GREAT CHEF? NOT TO WORRY!

You don't need to be a good cook to prepare the soup. You don't need to know how to cook at all. All you need to do is read and follow the simple directions that follow.

Important: The recipe below makes about 6 quarts of soup. If you do not own a pot large enough to accommodate all the ingredients, do yourself a favor and get one. In the meantime, you can easily halve the recipe by using only half of the amount of each ingredient.

It takes almost two hours to make the full recipe of the soup. This estimate includes approximately twenty minutes to clean and chop the vegetables, about half an hour for the soup to come to a boil, and about an hour of simmering to cook the vegetables and bring out their flavors.

Cabbage Soup

To make the soup, you'll need:

- 1 head white cabbage, outer leaves removed
- 6 large carrots, peeled
- 6 medium onions, peeled
- 6 green onions (scallions)
- 2 green or red sweet peppers
- 3 large whole tomatoes, or 1 28-ounce can whole tomatoes
- 5 stalks celery
- 2 cloves garlic, peeled
- 1½ cups uncooked brown rice
- Salt and pepper to taste
  (See chapter 9 for how to vary the flavor with low- or no-cal herbs, spices, and other flavoring ingredients.)

1. Slice the cabbage and other vegetables into bite-size pieces. If you are using whole canned tomatoes, slice these into bite-size pieces, too. Crush or mince garlic.
2. Place cabbage and other vegetables in a large pot and add about 6 quarts cold water.
3. Boil for 10 minutes uncovered, then cover the pot and simmer over low heat until vegetables are tender. (Some dieters like to bring out even more intense vegetable flavor by simmering the soup for longer periods.)
4. While the soup is simmering, cook 1½ cups brown rice according to package directions. Add cooked rice to soup when the soup is almost finished.
5. Add salt and pepper to taste when the soup is fully cooked.

That's it! Now you have a supply of great-tasting basic cabbage soup. Store it in the fridge and heat it up on the stove or in the microwave as needed.

How many servings does the recipe make, and how long will the soup last? That's up to you. Enjoy as much of it as you like, as often as you like, throughout the diet cycle. (You may be surprised at how quickly it disappears!)

CHAPTER 5

Free Vegetables, Free Fruits, Free Fish and Chicken

To lose the greatest number of pounds in seven days, you will have to follow the New Cabbage Soup Diet exactly as written. This means you will need to shop ahead of time so that you'll have enough of the right foods when you need them. You'll need to know which vegetables and fruits qualify as "free" varieties—the ones you can enjoy in un-limited amounts. And of those free vegetables and fruits, you'll need to know how to select the ones that deliver the best nutrition and the most delicious and satisfying flavors.

WHEN AND HOW TO SHOP FOR THEM

The day before you start the New Cabbage Soup Diet is the day to shop for much of what you will need. If you're planning to use mainly fresh vegetables and fruits, most will keep in the refrigerator from two to five days, and you will begin to use them almost immediately. Shop accordingly.

Buy a large and varied assortment initially. Only you can estimate the quantities, but a good rule of thumb is to take home just a little more than you think you will need, but not so much more that the fruits and vegetables will deteriorate before you get around to eating them. Shop again on Day 3 or 4, if necessary, so that you will have enough on hand to finish the diet cycle.

PICK OF THE CROP I: BEST NEW CABBAGE SOUP DIET VEGETABLES

The United States Department of Agriculture is the ultimate expert on shopping for vegetables and fruits. The agency offers these general pointers on buying the best:

- As a rule, the freshest vegetables offer the best nutritional value. Freshness in vegetables is indicated by bright color, crispness, and firmness.
- Don't buy just because the price is low. Although most produce is priced lowest when in season and theoretically at its best, low price sometimes goes hand in hand with deterioration and poor quality.
- Avoid partially decayed produce no matter how low the cost. Even if you are able to trim off the bad parts, deterioration will spread rapidly to the salvaged areas.

The vegetables on the list below are all "free" vegetables, meaning that you can have them in unlimited amounts on Days 2, 3, 6, and 7 of the New Cabbage Soup Diet. They're all low in calories and high in valuable nutrients. Vegetables not on the list have been omitted because they are too high in calories to be useful on the diet.

Important: When you make a shopping list, be sure to include the vegetables you will need for the cabbage soup:

1 head cabbage
6 large carrots
6 medium onions
6 green onions (scallions)
2 green or red sweet peppers
3 large whole tomatoes, or 1 28-ounce can whole tomatoes
5 stalks celery
2 cloves garlic

Now select as many different vegetables as you like from the following list. Choose a variety of leafy green vegetables; they'll help boost the calcium content of the diet. Also choose bright yellow, orange, and red vegetables, which are high in vitamin A and carotenoids.

The list includes shopping tips for potatoes. However, potatoes are not free vegetables; you may have only one on Day 2 of the diet.

Artichokes (1 medium, 60 calories) Look for plump, globe-shape artichokes that are heavy for their size. The leaves (more correctly called scales) should be compact and not widely spread, thick, green, and fresh looking. Avoid artichokes with spreading leaves (an indication of toughness and dryness), areas of brown or grayish discoloration, and mold growth. *Note:* Steamed artichoke leaves seasoned with a little lemon juice are good for nibbling anytime.

Asparagus (6 medium spears, 22 calories) The tips of asparagus should be closed and compact, and the spears should be round, smooth and green almost to the ends. Avoid tips that are open or spread out and "ribbed" spears; both indicate age and toughness.

Beans, green (½ cup, sliced, 22 calories) The best are firm and crisp with a bright green color. Avoid wilted, flabby beans, and those with thick, fibrous pods.

Beets (½ cup, sliced, 37 calories) Choose beets that are firm and round with a slender main root and deep red color over most of the surface. When beets are sold in a bunch with the tops still on, look for leaves that are fresh and in good condition. Avoid very large, misshapen beets, wilted or soft specimens, and those with scaly surface areas.

Broccoli (1 medium stalk, 50 calories) Look for compact, closed buds. The color of fresh, top-quality broccoli can range from dark, rich green to sage green, to green with a purplish cast. Avoid yellowish-green broccoli, buds that are enlarged or open, and specimens with soft or slippery spots on the bud clusters.

Brussels sprouts (½ cup, 30 calories) The freshest and best are a bright green in color, firm, and have tight-fitting outer leaves. Avoid soft sprouts and those with loose, wilted outer leaves.

Cabbage (1 cup, shredded or sliced, 33 calories) Smooth-leaved white cabbage is sold as new cabbage and storage cabbage. (The latter is grown in the fall and held for winter sale.) Select the firmest heads. Leaves should be reasonably free of blemishes. Outer leaves, called "wrapper leaves," are typically loose. Avoid wilted or yellow leaves and specimens with many loose wrapper leaves; they're waste, as you will be discarding them before you cook the cabbage. Storage cabbage is of a paler green color and usually trimmed of outer leaves. Avoid specimens with dried or discolored areas and those with outer leaf stems that have separated from the central stem at the base. As for red cabbage, the calorie count is approximately the same and so are the shopping tips.

Carrots (½ cup, sliced, 35 calories) Select bright orange, smooth, crisp, well-formed carrots. Avoid soft, flabby specimens.

Cauliflower (½ cup flowerets, 14 calories) Look for white or creamy white solid, clean "curds" (the white portion). Avoid softened, wilted, or discolored specimens and those with a smudgy or speckled appearance.

Celery (1 cup, sliced, 19 calories) Buy solid, glossy-looking, crisp stalks, light to medium green in color. Leaflets should be fresh looking or only slightly wilted. Avoid celery with soft or flabby upper stalks. Celery that is less than firm and crisp can be freshened slightly by placing cut stalks in water, but this procedure won't revive badly wilted celery.

Cucumbers (7 slices, 4 calories) Shop for cucumbers that are uniformly green and firm. Avoid very large cukes. Withered or shriveled ends signify toughness and bitter flavor.

Greens, leafy (1 cup, broken or chopped, about 15 calories. This is an average; different varieties deliver somewhat fewer or more calories) Vegetables in this group include spinach, kale, endive, escarole, chard, cress, chicory, and sorrel as well as collard, turnip, beet, mustard, and dandelion greens. Select leaves that are fresh, tender, and free from defects. Avoid wilted, soft or tough leaves, leaves with a yellowish-green cast, or thick, fibrous stems.

Lettuces (1 cup, pieces, approximately 8 calories; different varieties may contain somewhat fewer or more calories). All lettuces, including iceberg, Bibb, Boston, and romaine, should have fresh, blemish-free leaves. Iceberg and romaine leaves should be crisp. Other varieties have softer leaves.

Mushrooms (½ cup, sliced, 9 calories) Look for young, small- to medium-size mushrooms. In the freshest mushrooms, the cap is closed and the gills (the rows of paper-thin tissue under the cap) are not visible. When gills show, they should be pinkish or light tan. Avoid older mushrooms with pitted or discolored caps and dark brown or black gills.

Onions (1 cup, sliced, 60 calories; green onions or scallions, 1 cup chopped, 32 calories) Select mature onions that are firm and dry with a flat (not protruding) "neck." Avoid sprouted onions and those with wet or soft spots. Green onions should have fresh, crisp green tops. Avoid green onions with wilted or discolored tops.

Parsley (½ cup, chopped, 11 calories) Look for fresh, crisp, bright green leaves. Slightly wilted parsley can be freshened by trimming the stems and placing them in cold water in the refrigerator. Avoid yellowed or discolored leaves.

Peppers, sweet (1 cup strips, 22 calories) Choose glossy, firm, bright-colored specimens. The best are heavy relative to their size. Avoid peppers that "give" when pressed with a fingertip as well as those with moist surface areas.

Potatoes (1 medium baked, without skin, 145 calories) Potatoes are not free vegetables on the New Cabbage Soup Diet. You will be having only one white potato per seven-day cycle, but you may as well look for the best. Select a firm, smooth potato free of blemishes and "sunburn" (a green discoloration visible on or just under the skin). Avoid sprouted, withered, or bruised specimens.

Radishes (10 medium, 8 calories) Medium-size radishes, ¾ inch to 1 inch in diameter, are best. Look for plump, firm, bright red specimens. Avoid oversized, soft radishes and those with yellowed tops.

Summer squash (½ cup cooked, 18 calories) Summer squash varieties, including crookneck, zucchini, and patty pan, are harvested while still immature, when the entire squash is tender and edible. Some are available all year long. Buy glossy, firm, fresh-looking specimens. Avoid squash with dull, pitted, or toughened skin.

Tomatoes (1 2½-inch diameter uncooked, 26 calories; 1 cup, chopped, 38 calories) For best flavor, buy locally grown tomatoes, which usually are allowed to ripen on the vine. The most delectable tomatoes aren't always the most beautiful, perfectly symmetrical ones, but they should be blemish free and well ripened. A slight softness detectable by gentle pressure is an indication of ripeness. Avoid very soft or bruised tomatoes and those with moist areas or cracks on the surface. *Note:* If only underripe tomatoes are available, place them in a warm area away from direct sunlight for further ripening. (Cold temperatures delay ripening, so don't store them in the fridge.)

Turnips (½ cup cooked, 14 calories) The most widely available turnips have white flesh and a purple top. Buy small- or medium-size turnips that are smooth, firm, and globelike in shape. Avoid blemished or very large turnips; the latter tend to be tough and fibrous.

PICK OF THE CROP II: BEST NEW CABBAGE SOUP DIET FRUITS

No single fruit is a must on the New Cabbage Soup Diet. You can have as many different free fruits and as much as you like of any of them on Days 1, 3, and 7 of the diet.

Important: The following list includes shopping tips for bananas. However, bananas are not a free fruit and should be eaten only on Day 4 of the diet.

The general rules for selecting vegetables apply as well to fruits:

- The freshest fruits offer the best nutritional value. Bright, fresh color is one good indicator of freshness.
- Fruit that is unusually low in price is not always a bargain. Although prices tend to be lowest when the fruit is in season and most plentiful, don't forget that damage and overripeness also drive the price down.
- Don't buy fruit with signs of decay no matter how low the price. Even if you are able to trim off the bad areas, deterioration will spread quickly to salvaged areas.

Remember, with the exception of bananas, only the following fruits qualify as free fruits on the New Cabbage

Soup Diet. Don't eat fruits that are not on the list; some fruits have been excluded because they are too high in calories to qualify as "free."

Apple (1 medium, 2¼-inch diameter, 81 calories)   Of the many varieties of apples, some of the best for eating fresh are Delicious, McIntosh, Granny Smith, Empire, and Golden Delicious. Look for crisp, bright-colored apples with shiny skin. Avoid bruised and overripe apples. (These "give" easily with gentle pressure.) Apples with small tan or brownish spots are okay if the rest of the skin is smooth, firm, and shiny.

Apricots (1 medium, 17 calories)   Look for plump, juicy-looking fruit with a uniform, golden-orange color. Ripe apricots yield to gentle pressure. Avoid very soft or mushy fruit (too old) and very firm, pale- or greenish-yellow specimens (immature).

Bananas (1 medium, 104 calories)   Important: Bananas are not "free" on the New Cabbage Soup Diet; you'll be having them on Day 4 only. Shop for firm, bright yellow bananas with intact skin. Bananas are at their peak of flavor when tiny brown specks begin to appear on the skin. Bananas with green tips or skin that has not reached the bright yellow stage will ripen in a day or so after you get them home. Avoid bananas with advanced freckling or bruised or cracked skin.

Berries, including blackberries, boysenberries, loganberries, raspberries (1 cup, approximately 65 calories)   Although these berries are different in size and color, shopping guidelines are the same for all. Select berries that are bright-colored, clean, plump, and tender but not mushy. Avoid "leaky" berries (wet or stained areas on the carton indicate that the berries within are overripe or damaged) and berries with traces of mold or decay.

Blueberries (1 cup, 81 calories) Choose blueberries that are plump, firm, uniform in size, and of a dark blue color with a silvery bloom. Avoid soft, mushy, or leaking berries.

Cantaloupe (½ medium, 93 calories) Check for these signs of ripeness: a smooth, shallow scar where the stem used to be, thick netting or veining across some or all of the exterior, a yellowish-gray or pale yellow color under the netting. A ripe cantaloupe has a pleasant characteristic aroma and yields slightly to light pressure. Avoid over-ripeness, indicated by advanced softening of the rind.

Cherries (10 medium, 38 calories) Look for glossy, plump cherries with very dark color—from deep maroon to mahogany to almost black, depending on the variety. (Ranier cherries, which are straw-colored, are the exception.) Avoid shriveled or discolored cherries. Small areas of decay are hard to see against the dark color, so check carefully.

Grapefruit (½ medium, 38 calories) Pick firm, smooth-skinned specimens that are heavy for their size. Avoid grapefruit with very thick skin (signaled by a pebbly, rough, or crinkled surface). Soft, moist areas on the skin and skin that breaks with gentle finger pressure are signs of decay.

Grapes (10 medium, 35–40 calories, depending on the variety) Choose plump grapes that are firmly attached to their stems. As a general rule, bright characteristic color is an indicator of sweetness. Avoid soft, wrinkled, or leaking grapes and those with very brittle stems.

Honeydew (1 medium slice—about ¹⁄₁₀ melon, 45 calories) Shop for melons with a smooth, velvety surface, slightly softer at the blossom end, and a pleasant honeydew aroma. Avoid melons with no "give" (they're not quite ripe yet) and those with moist areas on the skin.

Kiwifruit (1 medium, 46 calories)   Look for plump, un-wrinkled fruit, light to medium greenish brown in color. Ripe fruit yields to gentle pressure; firm specimens are not quite ripe but will be ready to eat in a day or so if left at room temperature. Avoid wrinkled, shrunken kiwis.

Lemons (1 medium, about 17 calories; 1 tablespoon lemon juice, about 4 calories)   The best lemons are a rich, yellow color with smooth rather than pebbly skin. Pale, greenish-yellow lemons tend to be especially acidic. Avoid speci-mens with darker yellow or dull skin, signs of age that indicate a dryer, less juicy lemon.

Nectarines (1 medium, 67 calories)   Selec' plump, richly colored nectarines that have begun to soften slightly along the "seam." Hard, immature nectarines usually ripen at room temperature in two or three days. Avoid soft, overripe fruits and those with cracked or bruised skin.

Oranges (1 medium, about 62 calories)   Oranges are re-quired by law to be mature when harvested, thus a greenish cast or green spots do not indicate immaturity. Buy firm, smooth-skinned oranges that are heavy for their size. Avoid lightweight oranges, which may be short on juice and flesh. Rough, pebbly skin is often an indicator of dry, fibrous flesh. Dull, dry skin and a spongy consistency are signs of age and deteriorating quality.

Peaches (1 medium, 37 calories)   Ripe peaches will have velvety smooth skin and yield to gentle pressure. Underripe peaches will ripen at room temperature in a day or two after purchase. Avoid soft, mushy, or bruised specimens.

Pineapple (1 cup chunks, 76 calories)   Look for bright, golden yellow to reddish-brown pineapples with a pleasant, characteristic aroma and very slight lifting of the "eyes," or pips, on the rind. Avoid green, unripened pineapples as well as those with discolored, soft, or moist areas.

Plums (1 medium, 36 calories) Select deep or bright-colored plums that yield slightly to gentle pressure. Avoid hard, wrinkled, or mushy fruits.

Strawberries (1 cup whole medium berries, 45 calories) Choose bright red berries with lustrous skin, firm flesh with attached stem caps. Medium to small ripe strawberries often have richer, sweeter flavor than the giant-size ones. Avoid leaky strawberries and those with large colorless areas.

Tangerines (1 2¼-inch diameter, 37 calories) Lustrous, deep yellow to orange tangerines are best. Pale or greenish specimens may be less flavorful (however, small green areas on otherwise high-colored fruit are okay). The loose-fitting skin of a ripe tangerine yields to gentle pressure; this lack of firmness is not an indicator of poor quality. Avoid tangerines with soft, mushy surface areas.

Watermelon (1 cup chunks, 51 calories) If you are buying a slice of melon, choose one with firm, juicy, bright-red flesh, free of whitish streaks, and studded with dark brown or black seeds. Avoid melons with pale flesh and whitish seeds, which indicate the melon is not fully ripe. To judge the quality of a whole melon, look for smooth skin that is midway between shiny and matte. The ends of the melon should be filled out and rounded, not sunken, and the underside or belly of the melon should be creamy in color.

WHAT ABOUT FROZEN?

If you'd rather not shop every few days for fresh vegetables and fruit, go ahead, stock up on frozen. The calorie count and nutrient values of frozens are similar to those of fresh. Of course, any frozen vegetable or fruit you purchase should be frozen "plain"—with no syrup, no butter, no cream sauce or other seasoning or ingredient that boosts the calorie count. Frozen green beans are fine, for instance, but a frozen green bean and corn mix is not.

How to get top-quality frozen products: Examine the package. Don't buy frozen produce in packages that are limp, wet, or sweating; these conditions indicate that the contents are beginning to defrost. Stained packages and packages with ice clinging to them may have been defrosted and refrozen on the way from processor to supermarket. Although they should be safe to eat, they may not be as tasty as never-defrosted produce.

WHAT ABOUT CANNED?

Yes, use canned produce if you prefer. Canned vegetables and fruits are about the same as fresh or frozen in terms of calories and nutrients, but may not be as good tasting. (An exception is canned tomatoes. The flavor of canned tomatoes is very different from that of fresh, but it's a good flavor in its own right.)

When buying canned vegetables and fruit, read labels carefully. Avoid products canned with syrup or other ingredients that add calories.

SHOPPING FOR LOWEST-FAT CHICKEN AND FISH

The New Cabbage Soup Diet allows unlimited amounts of chicken or fish on Days 5 and 6. For optimal results, get the kind that is lowest in fat.

Chicken

As a rule, the younger the chicken, the less fatty it is. You can't very well ask about the age of individual chickens at the supermarket, but you don't have to. The youngest chickens are the smallest.

Smaller broilers and fryers are leaner than larger ones and have less fat than chickens sold for roasting. Even small chickens, though, have hunks of yellow fat inside. Cut away or tear off the fat before you cook the bird.

Fish

Fish is lower in fat than most other foods of animal origin, but some species have less fat than others. The least fatty fish are the species that have the whitest flesh.

White-fleshed, Lowest-fat Fish
Catfish
Haddock
Halibut
Scrod

Medium-fleshed, Medium-fat Fish
Bluefish
Catfish
Tuna

Darker-fleshed, Higher-fat Fish
Mackerel
Salmon
Swordfish

Avoid these higher-fat varieties for now.

What about Canned Tuna?

Obviously, fish from the white-fleshed, lowest-fat group are the best choices while you're blitzing off pounds on the New Cabbage Soup Diet. However, if you love tuna, a medium-fat fish, go ahead and enjoy it on Days 5 and 6 of the diet. Just make sure to buy the kind packed in water.

A LOOK AHEAD

You won't have to remember how much of each kind of food to eat on the New Cabbage Soup Diet. Chapters 11 through 17 contain food plans, what-to-eat reminders, plus tips and suggestions for each day of the diet. Be sure to read those chapters as you follow the diet.

• • •

Successful weight loss is more than just a physical process. It involves beliefs and attitudes, too. Don't skip the following chapter. It will help you prime your mind for dieting. In fact, it could make the difference between struggling to lose pounds and inches and easy, almost effortless weight loss.

CHAPTER 6

Priming Your Mind for Weight-Loss Success

The New Cabbage Soup Diet is easy to follow. It's made up of nutritious, great-tasting, low-calorie and low-fat foods to generate the quickest weight loss possible. It's a structured plan; you don't ever have to decide what or how much to eat because the entire diet is laid out for you in advance. And you can have unlimited amounts of many of the foods you will be eating, so hunger won't be a problem.

This diet gives you quick results and early, tangible signs of success. These signs—a significant drop in pounds, not to mention a trimmer-looking body, a new sense of lightness and well-being, and a new bounce to your step—generate the motivation you need to stay on track. As the diet quickly and efficiently rids your body of excess fat, you're going to feel more upbeat and confident about achieving your weight goal than you've felt on any diet you've ever tried in the past.

COMMITMENT IS THE KEY

But to lose every pound you want to lose, you must bring something to the table, too. That something is commitment. Motivation will come soon enough after you begin the diet. But commitment must exist from the very beginning.

Of course, you want to lose weight. If it wasn't high on your list of priorities, you wouldn't be reading this book.

But *wanting* to lose weight is not quite the same as *being committed* to losing weight.

For instance, you might really *want* to lose weight, but perhaps you've tried so many times in the past that achieving your goal seems like an elusive and impossible dream.

Or maybe you *want* to lose weight, but you've never done anything about it because you've heard so much about how hard it is from other dieters.

Or maybe you want to lose weight, but your real reason for going on a diet is to put a stop to the nagging you get from other people—your wife or husband, your kids, your doctor, maybe even your boss.

When you are full of doubts or your heart really isn't in it, you are not truly committed to the weight-loss process. And when that is the case, following a diet—any diet, including the New Cabbage Soup Diet—is more difficult than it needs to be.

If you want to lose weight, but your diet history—or other people—keep telling you how hard it is, or if your motives come from outside instead of within yourself, the techniques in this chapter can strengthen your commitment and turn your desire for a healthier, more attractive body into reality.

TAKE OUT A CONTRACT FOR SUCCESS

There is emotional commitment and there is contractual commitment, but in any kind of commitment there is always a promise, implied or explicit. When you commit yourself to another person, as in marriage, you promise to do certain things and not to do other things. When you commit yourself to buying a house, you promise to honor the terms of sale. When your application for a credit card is accepted, you promise to fulfill the obligations set out by the bank.

A genuine commitment to losing weight also involves a promise—in this case, a promise you make to yourself to abide by the terms of the weight-loss plan. But rather than simply "think" the promise, get it down on paper. Yes, put it in writing for the world to see. That way, your agreement with yourself becomes more real, more binding, more important than the silent promise that exists only in your mind. In fact, psychologists have found that a written contract is an effective tool for helping dieters and others keep the promises they make to themselves. Some believe that drawing up such a contract is an important predictor of success.

The most useful contract for you as a dieter will specify exactly what you intend to do and include small rewards or incentives at intervals along the way to the big payoff—which is, of course, achieving your weight-loss goal. It is also helpful to have the contract "witnessed" by a relative or friend. Here's a model contract for you to use:

Weight Loss Contract: Agreement Made with Myself

Beginning on _____ (*fill in starting date*), I
will eat in accordance with the New Cabbage Soup Diet
until _____ (*give ending date, seven days
later*).

I will give myself a small reward of one of the following
_____
(*enter three or four small nonfood treats*) at the end of
each day on the diet.

_____ (*name of
spouse, other relative, or friend*) has read and will sign
this contract.

_____

(*your signature*)

_____

(*signature of spouse, relative, or friend*)

PICK YOUR PRIZES

The reward you choose to give yourself at the end of every
successful New Cabbage Soup Diet day should be something pleasurable that you won't want to miss—something
that you will look forward to so much it will help you stay
on track throughout the day. The thought of even a small
treat can keep you going, especially if the treat is something

you don't ordinarily give yourself permission to enjoy.

A few ideas to start you thinking:

- Give yourself a long, luxurious bubble bath or do-it-yourself facial.
- Slip out to a movie, or watch that video you've been wanting to see.
- An uninterrupted half hour with a good book is a great reward if you love to read but rarely make the time for it.
- If you have access to a pool and enjoy swimming, a half hour in the water might be a great treat.
- Maybe just visiting with friends or having free time all to yourself would be enough.

If you are the parent of small children, you may need co-operation from your spouse, another adult, or a babysitter to enjoy rewards like these, but asking for help, and even paying for it if necessary, is worth it.

Giving yourself small rewards for every successful day on the New Cabbage Soup Diet is tantamount to "success insurance." In fact, it is so useful, the technique is included in each of the diet days chapters.

SELF-TALK, PEP TALK

Another technique for strengthening your commitment to this diet—or to achieving any worthwhile goal—is to talk to yourself in positive terms. Of course, you needn't actually talk aloud. Thinking the words is enough.

The basic idea is to rid your mind of negative thoughts and instill positive thoughts in their place. It also involves replacing negative phrases—such as "I'll never be able to see this through," or "Stupid me, here I go again on another diet that's not going to help me"—with positive phrases like "I *will* follow this diet," or "I *know* I'll be successful this time."

The self-talk technique draws on some of the principles

of cognitive therapy. Practitioners of this form of therapy believe that feelings and behavior spring from words, and that what we say to ourselves and others greatly influences how we feel and what we do. According to cognitive therapists, anxiety, doubt, and even depression are in large part the result of using negative words and phrases in the continuing mental conversation we have with ourselves. The opposite is true as well. Feelings of confidence grow when we use positive words and phrases.

If you doubt the effectiveness of positive self-talk, try saying to yourself "I feel terrific!" a few times in the course of the next ten minutes. Say it with conviction and a smile on your face. Notice how your body begins to relax and your mood starts to lift.

Self-Talk Basics

- Among the negative phrases to watch out for are any that include "no," "not," "never," "can't," and "couldn't." When you are aware of having said words like these to yourself, correct them immediately with a contradictory positive statement. Change "I'm no good at sticking to a diet" to "I can stick to a diet." Change "I've never had any willpower" to "I do have willpower."

- Do the same when you realize you have been mentally downing yourself with phrases such as "I'm such a failure," "I'm incompetent," "I never get it right." Negative self-talk can create feelings of helplessness and hopelessness and does more than almost anything else to damage self-respect. Negative words and phrases also can deepen or lead to depression. And depression can make you vulnerable to the temptation to "self-medicate" the blues with food.

- As often as possible, use these same principles in conversation with other people. The negative words and phrases we use in referring to ourselves in company are just as potent as the ones we use in our private mental conversations. They may be even more damaging because in broadcasting doubts and anxieties about dieting (or anything else), we also define ourselves as "likely to fail" in the eyes of others.

Positive self-talk, like giving yourself a small reward at the end of each diet day, is so important, the concept is included in the diet chapters of this book—only instead of just pumping yourself up with positive thoughts, you'll also be writing them down in a journal.

FIND A CHEERLEADER

Some diet experts urge people who want to shape up to find a community of other dieters with whom to share feelings and experiences. The opportunity to meet regularly with other dieters for mutual support is offered by some of the major commercial weight-loss organizations and accounts for much of their success. Talking about the weight-loss process, freely and without embarrassment, has indeed proven useful to some dieters. But there is a downside to sharing diet thoughts and feelings: Not everyone has good news to report, and the bad news can be disheartening, especially to those who are just starting out on a new weight-loss program.

There's a better way to get help when you are starting a diet, and that is to find a "cheerleader"—one person who is upbeat, positive, and 100 percent on your side. If you know anyone who fits that description, spend some time with her or him before you begin the diet. Talk about what you want to accomplish and how you are going to do it. Ask for positive feedback.

A good candidate might be someone you know who is also about to start the New Cabbage Soup Diet. Ask around. There is more interest in the diet—and there are more people who want to lose weight—than you might imagine.

In any event, pick your cheerleader carefully, because some people may do more harm than good. Someone with a long history of diet failure may not be wholly supportive of your efforts. For obvious reasons, you also should avoid anyone with a sarcastic, cynical turn of mind.

OR KEEP IT TO YOURSELF
What if you don't connect with someone who will be fully supportive and with you all the way? If you think about the principles of self-talk—the value of positive words and phrases and the destructive power of negative words and phrases—you will understand why it is almost always better not to talk about your diet at all than to risk talking with people who put a negative spin on your efforts. In short, if you can't find a cheerleader, don't ask, don't tell is the best policy.

ONE DAY AT A TIME, PLEASE
The New Cabbage Soup Diet is meant to be followed for just one week (three days if you want to blitz off just two or three pounds). At the end of the week, you'll have to decide among several options. You can switch to a good, long-term diet (if you want to lose more weight). You can create your own healthful, well-balanced food plan with the suggestions in chapter 18. Or you can move on to the Cabbage Soup Maintenance Plan, outlined in chapter 19. And, of course, you can return to the New Cabbage Soup Diet at any point along the way, assuming you allow at least two weeks to elapse between each seven-day cycle. Whatever you do, you'll be more successful if you maintain a strong commitment to a slimmer, fitter body.

One of the enemies of commitment, however, is the feeling of being overwhelmed by the magnitude of the task. We may begin to focus on all the time it will take, all the willpower we will have to exert, all the deprivations we must undergo. If we focus too much on these challenges, we may begin to wonder if it is within our power actually to accomplish what we set out to achieve, and this uncertainty can lead to procrastination or even to a decision to scrap the project. But even if we grit our teeth and decide to move forward, the feeling of being overwhelmed can make it harder than it needs to be, especially if we insist on thinking of the project as one big mountain we have to move.

But something almost miraculous happens when we mentally break the job into smaller pieces. Thinking one pound at a time or one day at a time can change our perspective and shift our focus in ways that make the project seem more manageable.

Think about it. Doesn't the idea of losing weight a pound at a time seem more achievable than the concept of losing, say, a hundred pounds? Doesn't thinking of staying on a diet one day at a time somehow feel more comfortable than thinking in terms of weeks, years, or the rest of our lives?

A big job always is accomplished in pieces, whether we view it that way or not. We write a lengthy report one page at a time. We paint a room one wall at a time. We lose weight one pound at a time, and we stay on a diet one day at a time. When we make a conscious, prior decision to break a project into smaller pieces, much of that feeling of being overwhelmed goes away—and along with it go many of the doubts we felt about our ability to achieve the goal.

The one-step-at-a-time technique is something like the techniques used in twelve-step programs and has helped thousands of alcoholics, drug users, and, yes, even dieters to move toward their goals. You will rarely, if ever, hear a recovering alcoholic who has attended twelve-step meetings say, "I'll never take another drink . . . ever." Or "liquor is no longer an option." Instead, she or he might say, "I choose not to have a drink now."

To benefit from the technique, focus your attention in the present moment—not on the mistakes you made yesterday or on the difficulties you might encounter tomorrow or the day after, and certainly not on the prospect of never again indulging in foods that are bad for you. If your attention begins to stray back to the past or forward into the future, rein it in. Command it to stay in the present, and see how much better it feels to live and control your weight in the here and now.

Commitment to the weight-loss process is the key to success on any diet. Now that you understand the commitment-strengthening techniques in this chapter, the key is in your hand. But, as you know, techniques such as these are just words on paper until you actually put them to work for you. So give them your best shot. Their usefulness may surprise you.

In the next chapter, which sets out the New Cabbage Soup Diet rules, you will find everything you need to know to be a winner at the losing game. Success depends on playing by these rules, so be sure to read it before you start the diet.

CHAPTER 7

Rules to Lose By

Yes, you can lose up to ten pounds—maybe even more!—
in your first seven-day cycle of the New Cabbage Soup
Diet, and you can lose up to five pounds on the three-day
blitz version. But only if you follow the rules.

It shouldn't be difficult. You'll never experience real
hunger on this diet because you can fill up on the soup as
often as you want to, whenever you want to. The food is
healthful, plentiful, and good tasting, as you will see when
you read chapter 9, there are many quick and easy ways to
make it even tastier and more satisfying.

Still, this diet has a more rigid structure than most other
weight-loss plans, and it's strict in the sense that you must
abide by certain rules.

It's going to demand a lot from you, but think of it this
way: The rules of the diet leave nothing to chance. You
can't make mistakes on the diet if you follow them exactly.
In fact, taken together, the rules provide your blueprint for
success.

Rule 1. Get a doctor's permission to start the diet.
Rule 2. Don't make food substitutions.
Rule 3. Don't omit foods.
Rule 4. Eat until you feel full and satisfied, then stop.
Rule 5. No alcohol.
Rule 6. Cook chicken and fish the lowest-fat way.

Rule 7. Have vegetables raw, steamed, or grilled.
Rule 8. Don't use calorie-laden condiments.

RULE 1. GET A DOCTOR'S PERMISSION TO START THE DIET

This is a prime rule no dieter should ignore. It was mentioned first in chapter 1 and is repeated here because it's so important. Be sure to explain to your doctor that you plan to use the diet for seven days only and that you will allow two weeks or more to elapse before you start a second cycle. While you are discussing the diet, ask the doctor if she or he thinks it would be a good idea for you to take a multivitamin and mineral supplement.

RULE 2. DON'T MAKE FOOD SUBSTITUTIONS

As you know, the New Cabbage Soup Diet is not just low in fat, it's also low in calories. Calorie consciousness is in accord with the latest thinking in nutrition; for weight loss to take place, it is as important to limit calories as it is to limit fat. That fact has been stressed throughout this book.

But despite the emphasis on calories in the New Cabbage Soup Diet, it doesn't follow that all calorically equal foods are equally good for effecting quick weight loss. Or that you can substitute food delivering equal numbers of calories for the foods specified on the diet and still achieve the same, speedy results.

For example, a ½-cup serving of fat-free frozen yogurt dessert provides approximately 140 calories. Two medium-size apples come in at about 162 calories. Knowing this, you might assume that there is no reason not to snack on a serving of the no-fat yogurt dessert—a "diet" food, after all—instead of the apples (or any of the other free fruits or vegetables on the diet). If you went with the yogurt dessert, you would even be "saving" 22 calories.

No one can dispute the 22-calorie savings, but that

doesn't compensate for the nutritional difference between apples and yogurt dessert. With the apples, you get vitamins and phytochemicals that contribute to your health and well-being. Just as important, the apples provide some fiber, which, according to many researchers, increases the amount of fat excreted by the body, and which certainly enhances feelings of fullness and satisfaction.

On the other hand, with fat-free frozen yogurt, you get approximately 15 grams of sugars in the form of ordinary refined sugar, corn syrup, and other sweeteners. Sugars like these don't advance the weight-loss process and therefore have no place on the New Cabbage Soup Diet. The frozen yogurt dessert won't keep you satisfied for very long—in fact, as with many other foods containing refined sugars, consuming it may trigger hunger for more. Where calcium is concerned, the frozen yogurt dessert has a nutritional advantage (a ½-cup serving supplies approximately 20 percent of the daily requirement). But you will be consuming that much calcium and more in the vegetables and the skim milk or plain, fat-free yogurt you'll be having every day of the diet.

The point, of course, is not to slam fat-free frozen yogurt desserts or any other food that is not part of the New Cabbage Soup Diet. There may be times when frozen yogurt dessert is an ideal snack or the perfect way to end a meal. But not when you are on this diet.

The same is true of dozens of other foods that are caloric equivalents of the foods specified on the New Cabbage Soup Diet—but that do nothing to speed the weight-loss process. It would take pages and pages to list all of these foods and explain why in each case you are better off avoiding them while you are on this diet. Having a blanket no-substitutions rule covers all bases. The surest, best way to get rid of unwanted pounds in a hurry is to abide by this no-substitutions rule and consume nothing that is not specifically mentioned as part of the diet.

RULE 3. DON'T OMIT FOODS

Every food on the New Cabbage Soup Diet is important.
You won't achieve the same quick results if you skip any
of them.

The cabbage soup is a low-calorie, high-nutrition food
that is rich in vitamins, phytochemicals, and fiber. Because
the soup can be eaten anytime and in unlimited amounts,
it's a sure-cure for hunger, should it ever arise.

Like the soup, the free vegetables and fruits supply important nutrients and fiber and act to block hunger by helping to keep blood sugar levels steady.

All those bananas on Day 4, when you are approximately halfway through the seven-day diet cycle, will help
you cope with carbohydrate cravings that might begin to
kick in at about that time. Bananas are important, too, because they provide a sweet change of pace and texture
while supplying you with fair amounts of vitamin A, niacin
and iron, some protein, and an abundance of potassium.

The chicken or fish on Days 5 and 6 boosts the protein
content of the diet.

All the different elements of the New Cabbage Soup
Diet, and the way they work together, will keep you feeling
satisfied, keep food cravings to a minimum, and, most important, get rid of the pounds you want to lose. You won't
get the same, extraordinary results if you skip any of them.

RULE 4. EAT UNTIL YOU FEEL FULL AND SATISFIED, THEN STOP

Rule 3 tells you to have some of every food included on
the diet, but Rule 4 reminds you that this is not a com-
mandment to fill up on enormous amounts of any of them.

For example, you must eat at least one serving of cabbage soup every day you are on the diet, and you also are
encouraged to use the soup as a hunger-blocker between
meals or whenever you feel the need to eat something. But
you are not required to eat huge amounts of the soup to
keep the weight-loss process on track. Have as much as

you want, but if one or two bowls a day are enough to make you feel comfortably full, there is no need to eat more.

It's the same with the bananas on Day 4 and the chicken or fish on Days 5 and 6. Have as much as it takes to make you feel comfortably satisfied, but don't eat just because the food is available to you.

How much of the free vegetables and fruits you eat is entirely up to you. You should have several servings on days when they are part of the diet, but you don't have to consume enormous quantities.

You will lose pounds and inches on this unique diet no matter how much cabbage soup and free vegetables and fruits it takes to fill you up. But you probably will feel full and satisfied on smaller amounts of these foods than you think now.

RULE 5. NO ALCOHOL

Alcohol is not permitted on the New Cabbage Soup Diet. From "lite" beer to vodka, all alcoholic beverages contain unnecessary and "empty" calories.

An equally important reason to avoid alcohol on this or any diet has to do with its capacity to lower inhibitions. Even a single drink might relax your inhibitions and cloud your judgment enough to interfere with your commitment to losing weight. Next thing you know, you might be sipping a second drink—accompanied by handfuls of nachos and guacamole.

It is a good idea to avoid parties and other events where alcohol is served during the seven-day diet cycle. When you must make an appearance, ask for sparkling water or seltzer with ice and a wedge of lemon or lime. (Seltzer is calorie-free and, unlike club soda, contains no salt.) These refreshing alternatives will give you something to do with your hands and will not dull the part of your brain that keeps you alert and motivated to stay on the diet.

RULE 6. COOK CHICKEN AND FISH THE LOWEST-FAT WAY

Where chicken and fish are concerned, there are two things to consider. One is the fat content of the item itself. The other is the method of cooking. In chapter 5, you learned which types of chicken and fish are lowest in fat. Here we're concerned with how to cook them.

First, do not use fat in preparing these items. Cooking fat adds unnecessary calories. For instance, a tablespoon of corn, peanut, or olive oil has 124 calories, and even though the oil is used only as a cooking medium, some of those extra calories will end up in your stomach. It's the same with butter, at 102 calories per tablespoon.

Grilling, broiling, roasting, steaming, and poaching are all excellent no-fat ways to cook chicken or fish, the two "meat" items on this diet.

- *Grilling.* Grilling is quick, easy if you have the right equipment, and imparts uniquely delicious flavor. In grilling, food is cooked *above* the heat source; fat, if any, is melted by the heat and drips down between the rods of the grill rack. In effect, this method not only requires no fat, it also defats the food as it cooks.

Canadian Rule for Grilling or Broiling Fish to Perfection

It's simple. Just cook the fish 10 minutes for every inch of thickness. You'll know it's done when the flesh turns from translucent to opaque and flakes slightly when you test it with a fork.

- *Broiling.* In broiling, food is cooked below the heat source. It's as quick and easy as grilling, but unless you take precautions, fat liquefied during cooking will pool around the item and may soak into it. To elevate fish or chicken out of any liquefied fat, broil on a rack. (*Note:* A rack will lift the food closer to the heat source, so adjust the position of the broiler rack, if necessary, to avoid burning the food.)

- *Roasting.* Another method of cooking food without added fat, roasting is done in the oven, usually at temperatures of around 325°F. Roasting typically takes longer than grilling and broiling. Use this method for chicken, if you like, but don't attempt to roast fish. In roasting, liquefied fat can accumulate in the roasting pan and soak into the underside of the chicken. You can avoid this by roasting the chicken on a rack placed in the roasting pan.
- *Steaming and poaching.* These are less popular ways of cooking fish and chicken without added fat, but they are certainly worth considering. Steaming or poaching fish is especially good since these methods produce a wonderfully delicate flavor and a flaky consistency that are hard to duplicate through other cooking methods. There are special utensils designed for steaming and poaching fish. If you don't own a fish steamer/poacher, you can obtain similar results by steaming in an inch or so of water (or cabbage soup liquid!) in a covered skillet. Add a few leaves of crushed fresh herbs for even more flavor. Check frequently for doneness, and add more liquid if necessary. Cooking time will depend on the thickness of the fish.

Chicken breasts can be poached in the same way. Place them in a covered skillet in 1½ inches of simmering water. Cover the pan and check for doneness after 10 minutes or so. Add more liquid as necessary. (Cooking time will vary depending on the thickness of the chicken breast.)

RULE 7. HAVE VEGETABLES RAW, STEAMED, OR GRILLED

Like Rule 5, this one helps keep the fat content of the diet as low as possible.

- *Raw* veggies, of course, need practically no preparation. Just scrub, dry, and slice into bite-size pieces. Keep a selection in the refrigerator so they will be available whenever you want something crunchy and good tasting on the diet days when unlimited vegetables are permitted. You also can have a selection of raw vegetables, or crudités, as part of a meal. Serve with lemon juice or a dip of plain, no-fat yogurt sprinkled with fresh chives, dill, or other fresh herbs.

> *Note:* Scientists now recognize that cooking actually adds to the nutritional value of some vegetables, especially those that are high in fiber.
>
> Fiber can "trap" phytochemicals in vegetables, making them less available to the body. Heat, on the other hand, helps free up phytochemicals. As a general rule, cook vegetables until they are tender but not mushy, as overcooking can destroy some of the vitamin C.

- *Steaming* vegetables helps retain nutrients that might otherwise be leached out in boiling water. If you don't already have one, get a vegetable steamer that fits into a saucepan. To cook by steaming: Add an inch or so of water to the saucepan, insert the steamer, place the vegetables inside, and check to see that the water level is low enough not to submerge the veggies. Cook the vegetables until tender. Check frequently for doneness; steaming can be quicker than boiling!
- *Grilling* is a wonderful way to cook vegetables. The intense, direct heat caramelizes the natural sugars, adding delectable flavor. Although some cookbooks

suggest brushing a little oil on vegetables before placing them on the grill, you can also get excellent results without the oil. Check frequently to avoid
charring.
* *Microwaving* vegetables is convenient, quick, and a
good way to preserve nutrients. Follow instructions
in your microwave manual for how long and at what
setting to cook various vegetables.

RULE 8. DON'T USE CALORIE-LADEN CONDIMENTS

In chapter 9 you will find suggestions for enhancing the
flavor of many of the foods you will be eating on the New
Cabbage Soup Diet. Every flavoring tip in that chapter is
low in calories and low in fat. There are many other flavor
ingredients not listed there, and you might wonder about
them. It's impossible to list every flavoring or condiment
on the market, so read labels and follow these guidelines:

* Don't use condiments or flavorings that have more
than 25 calories per tablespoon.
* If a condiment or flavoring ingredient has fewer than
25 calories per tablespoon, you can use 1 tablespoon
of it once a day.
* If a condiment or flavoring ingredient has fewer than
5 calories per tablespoon, you can use as much of it
as you like.

Don't use "regular" bottled salad dressing. In this context, "regular" means that the dressing in question is *not*
labeled low fat or no fat. Regular dressings are made with
too much oil and deliver too many calories. Regular Rus-
sian dressing, for example, has approximately 76 calories
per tablespoon; many low-fat versions have about 4 calories
per tablespoon, so you can use them on the New Cabbage
Soup Diet to add more flavor to salads or vegetables. Unfortunately, classic oil and vinegar salad dressing, commercial and homemade—the kind many people prefer over

all others—has about 72 calories per tablespoon. Do not use it while you are on this diet.

Chapter 3 addressed the sugar vs. artificial sweetener question, but to reiterate: Say no to sugar; if you want to sweeten coffee or tea, use artificial sweetener.

Follow these simple rules and you'll be on track and headed for a visibly slimmer, trimmer body in less time than you ever thought possible. Remember, this diet is strict, but it's not hard to follow. You will have to pay attention to everything you eat, but you'll be enjoying plenty of good-tasting, healthful food—in fact, you will be eating more than enough to keep you feeling full and satisfied.

CHAPTER 8

Ten Bonus Tips for Optimal Results

Now you know the rules of the diet and why they are so important. Don't break or even bend the rules. Think of them as iron-clad—the Eight Commandments of rapid weight loss on the New Cabbage Soup Diet. Success depends on following them to the letter.

The tips and suggestions in this chapter are different. They're not essential to losing pounds and inches, but they *can* make the weight loss even easier. In fact, some of these tips are so useful, they'll be repeated again and again in chapters 11 through 17, the "diet days" chapters that walk you step-by-step through the entire seven-day cycle.

Much of what follows is based on work done by weight-control experts and psychologists looking for ways to help people lose the excess pounds that threaten their health and make their lives less joyful. Other tips and suggestions grew out of the experience of successful dieters who discovered through trial and error that certain approaches were helpful to them in achieving their goals while other approaches seemed to make dieting more difficult.

Read them all. Make a special note of the tips that seem most relevant to you and the circumstances of your life.

TIPS FOR TAKING OFF
1. Keep a diet journal.
2. Pick a convenient time to start the diet.

3. Shop ahead.
4. Don't overeat the day before you start the diet.
5. Whenever possible, have meals alone or with close family members only.
6. Decide how to handle family meals.
7. Pack a lunch on workdays.
8. Know what to order in restaurants.
9. Be more active.
10. Keep going, even if you slip.

1. Keep a Diet Journal

This might be the most important tip of all.

You'll need a journal to keep the facts straight. For instance, you'll be recording your starting weight and measurements in your journal so that you'll know at the end of the seven-day cycle—or three-day cycle if you're using the blitz version—just how many pounds and inches you've lost.

But your diet journal should be more than just a record-keeping device. It also should be be a motivating tool—as useful to you in staying committed to your goal as the positive self-talk discussed in chapter 6. Actually, writing in your diet journal is a form of self-talk, made visible in ink or pencil, in which you reaffirm your intention to stick to the rules of the diet, tell yourself that you are in control of your eating, and cheer yourself on.

There may be times during the diet when you feel a little shaky about your resolve, times when you are tempted to eat a favorite food that is not part of the diet, times when you don't feel at all confident about your ability to stay on track. Never mind. Write as if you believe.

As with positive self-talk, the strong, positive words and phrases you use in your diet journal have a power of their own. Those words and phrases will affect your feelings, and your feelings will affect your behavior. In a very real sense, the phrases you jot down in your diet journal will be self-fulfilling.

Of course, the kind of diet journal we're talking about

here is different from a diary in which you confess your failures, vent your anger and frustration, and air your deepest, darkest fears. Just as positive journal writing has the power to strengthen and motivate you, negative writing can undermine and weaken your resolve. However, it can be very helpful to write about close calls—times when you were tempted to chuck the diet and go on a high-calorie eating spree but didn't, for example. The fact that you resisted proves how strong and committed you are. That's something to feel good about and deserves to be recorded in your journal so you can refer back to your success when you need a shot of self-esteem.

In chapters 11 through 17, you will be urged to write a few lines in your journal twice a day, once in the morning soon after you wake up and again in the evening just before you turn in for the night.

2. Pick a Convenient Time to Start the Diet

With enough commitment, you can start the New Cabbage Soup Diet anytime, any day of the week. Still, you can make the whole process easier if you arrange to diet during a relatively quiet week when your schedule isn't cluttered with a round of social and business engagements where food and drink are part of the agenda.

If you're a veteran dieter, you already know how difficult it can be to navigate your way through the holidays— or even through a single party or business lunch—without being tempted to have at least a taste of food you know is incompatible with your weight-loss plan. It will be even more difficult while you are on the New Cabbage Soup Diet because of the way it's structured. Although this unique plan offers plenty of food and you'll never experience true hunger while you're on it, much of that food is different from the kind ordinarily served at a party or business lunch.

For some readers, the suggestion to pick a quiet week for dieting will seem impossible to carry out because you rarely have a quiet week. If that's your situation, and you really do want to lose pounds with this phenomenal quick

weight-loss plan, consider changing your schedule to fit the
diet instead of waiting to start the diet when your schedule
permits. With some advance planning, you should be able
to cancel or reschedule events that would otherwise interfere with diet success.

3. SHOP AHEAD

The importance of shopping ahead for the food you'll be
enjoying on the New Cabbage Soup Diet was discussed in
chapter 5, but it's worth repeating now, when you are gear-
ing up to start this amazing plan.

The day before Day 1 of the diet, make a list of all the
foods you will need for the entire seven-day cycle. (Do the
same if you plan to use the diet for three days.)

In making your list, be guided by the master diet plan
in chapter 3. Keep in mind that many fresh vegetables and
fruits begin to lose their freshness after two or three days
in the refrigerator, and buy accordingly.

Quantities and amounts are up to you. It's better, however, to buy a little more, rather than less, than you think
you will need. That way you won't have to run back to the
market when you suddenly realize the next day is a free
vegetable day, but all you have in the fridge is fruit.

4. Don't Overeat the Day Before You Start the Diet

You might have an impulse to binge the day before you
begin the diet. Many people do. It's almost as if the fact
that they are planning to diet tomorrow gives them license
to indulge in an orgy of eating today. ("Eat, drink, and be
merry, for tomorrow we shall diet!")

But resist that urge you must if you want to lose as much
weight as possible during the seven-day diet cycle. Over-
eating on the day before puts you at a real disadvantage
because your body will have to deal with the excess before
it can get down to the serious business of getting rid of
excess pounds.

You will lose pounds and inches no matter what you eat

the day before Day 1 on the New Cabbage Soup Diet, but you will lose more if you eat moderately on that day.

5. Whenever Possible, Have Meals Alone or with Close Family Members Only

Sounds unsociable, but you will be lowering your risk of straying off track if you can arrange to take most of your meals alone. That way you won't be tempted by what your tablemates are eating.

Almost as risky as watching others enjoy your favorites foods is listening to their mealtime comments. And, as you've probably noticed already, mealtimes almost always elicit comments about food and dieting—especially when the people you are eating with know that you are trying to lose weight.

You can never be sure that some well-meaning person, knowing that you are dieting, won't insist that you really don't need to lose weight and that you look fine just the way you are. Or that he or she won't urge you to taste something you shouldn't eat—"just a tiny taste, it's sooo delicious!" Or even attempt to seduce you into trying his or her own favorite weight-loss program. Comments like these aren't helpful and can be downright demoralizing. If you can't avoid other people at mealtimes, be prepared by steeling yourself in advance against temptation and discouragement.

Of course, you can hardly avoid your spouse, children, or roommates, so tell them about your diet before you get started. Explain what you want to accomplish during the week and ask for their help. "Help" in this sense simply means that they will not disparage your efforts or tempt you with foods that are not part of the New Cabbage Soup Diet.

6. Decide How to Handle Family Meals

A decision made early on can prevent confusion arising out of questions about who will cook what, as well as who will eat what.

Don't—repeat don't—try to impose this or any diet on the people you live with. You are the one who wants to lose weight. If other adults want to join you, that's fine, but it must be their decision.

As for children and teenagers, the New Cabbage Soup Diet, as you know, is not suitable for young, growing bodies and should not be used by anyone who has not reached physical maturity.

If you are the chief cook and meal planner at your house, it may be possible to integrate the diet with family meals simply by augmentation. Offer the cabbage soup as well as vegetables, fruit, chicken, or fish (depending on which day's plan you are following) to family members, but make sure there is plenty of other food for them to eat as well.

If someone else is the cook and meal planner, life will be simpler for everyone if *you* assume responsibility for your food so that others can cook and eat as they normally do.

The actual course you decide to follow here is less important than arriving at an agreement that encourages consistency and follow-through.

7. Pack a Lunch on Workdays

The New Cabbage Soup Diet was practically made for people on the job. Just ladle some soup into a plastic container, grab raw vegetables or fruit, cooked chicken or fish from the refrigerator, add napkins, spoon and fork, stow in a bag, and you're set. Assuming there is a microwave at work, warm the soup before you eat it. It's a fact that hot meals are more satisfying than cold.

8. Know What to Order in Restaurants.

The New Cabbage Soup Diet is not particularly restaurant-friendly. However, when you must dine out, you can always rely on the following:

- Green salad or plain vegetables on free vegetable days

- Fruit salad or plain fruit on free fruit days
- Broiled or grilled chicken or fish on Days 5 and 6

Think of these foods as your collective "ace in the hole" when you cannot avoid eating away from home. Even when they are not featured on the menu, most restaurants will accommodate your request for a portion of one of these foods and serve it to you plain, with no sauce or dressing.

When friends invite you to dinner, let them know in advance that you are following the New Cabbage Soup Diet and ask if you can have just a simple green salad, fruit salad, vegetables, or broiled chicken or fish. Good friends will be happy to cooperate. If there are reasons why they can't or won't, you can always bring your own food. (You won't be the first dieter in history who arrived at a party with dinner in hand.)

Of course, key your food choices to the day of the diet. To be sure which foods are appropriate for which days on the diet, double-check the menu for that day before you leave the house. On Day 1 you can have unlimited free fruit, but no vegetables, for example. On Day 5 you can have as much chicken or fish as you like, but no vegetables other than tomatoes, and no fruit.

9. Be More Active

No, it's not imperative that you embark on an all-out fitness program at the same time that you begin the diet. But now is a perfect time to begin to develop the habit of moving your muscles a little more, and a little more often, than you normally would. The benefits flowing from just a little more activity far outweigh the expenditure of time and energy.

Faster calorie burn-off is one of those benefits. Every move you make requires energy in the form of calories. A very small increase in activity, of course, burns only a very small numbers of calories, but over time the extra effort can make a difference.

The advantages of being more active don't stop there. Even a little bit of extra activity can help refresh and energize your body and your mind. It can help you refocus on your priorities. Many people have discovered that when they include a few minutes of physical activity in the morning, they are better prepared for challenges in the day ahead—including dieting challenges.

In each day of the day-by-day New Cabbage Soup Diet chapters that follow, you will find suggestions for being just a little more active. You will lose weight on the diet whether you act on these suggestions or not. But by increasing your activity level even slightly, you can insure that you will lose as much weight as it is possible to lose, and at the same time make the whole process easier.

10. Keep Going, Even If You Slip

Many dieters behave as if one slipup—a single ice-cream cone, a few French fries, a piece of buttered bread—can undo all the good that previous days of dieting have accomplished. Convinced that all is lost, they abandon the diet and return to their old way of eating. Worse, they decide that because they haven't been able to stick to a particular diet, they will never get rid of the weight they want to lose and, in a fit of self-loathing, they go off on a food binge.

Every word in this book was written to help make the New Cabbage Soup Diet so easy to follow you won't have to deal with slipups like these and the self-destructive behavior that often follows.

In the real world, of course, some people do give in to temptation and eat food that is not part of the diet. If that should happen to you, try to keep in mind that a single transgression does not wipe out the benefit of all your previous efforts.

Where weight loss is concerned, one day on the New Cabbage Soup Diet is better than no day at all. Two days are better still. And in every case, continuing with the diet after a slipup is better than abandoning it.

So don't be too hard on yourself if your commitment lapses and you go off track. Don't say to yourself "It's no use, I can't stay on the diet, so I might as well eat everything I want." If you really want to "punish" yourself for a small transgression, a better way to do it is to get right back on the diet.

It's almost time to begin. But before you do, take a look at the next chapter, telling how to give the New Cabbage Soup Diet more taste appeal. With the suggestions in that chapter fresh in your mind, you will be able to put more flavor into your meals and obtain maximum satisfaction along with maximum weight loss.

CHAPTER 9

Great Taste! How to Make It Even More Satisfying

You can follow the New Cabbage Soup Diet just as it was revealed in chapter 3. That would be the spartan approach. It's a perfectly good approach and one that has already helped thousands of dieters across the country lose the pounds that slowed them down, sapped their energy, made them look older, and increased their risk for a range of diseases.

Maybe you, too, prefer the no-frills spartan approach for its ease and simplicity. Maybe you don't particularly want to enjoy food while you are on a diet. Maybe you want to "take" food, like medicine, while you are on a diet. Lots of people feel the same way.

But if you are in the majority and don't want to subsist on plain food if there is an easy, tastier alternative, there is a different, much more flavorful approach.

You can make practically every food called for on the New Cabbage Soup Diet better tasting and more satisfying. You can do it in almost no time at all and with almost no extra effort. All it takes is some imagination, a few guidelines for creating new food combinations—and for using traditional combinations in untraditional ways—plus some no-calorie and super-low-calorie herbs, spices, and other seasonings.

TASTE APPEAL

If you decide to take the more flavorful and adventurous approach to New Cabbage Soup Dieting, you'll be amazed at the way certain combinations and certain ingredients, judiciously used, contribute to your enjoyment of the honest, wholesome but admittedly plain fare featured on the diet.

In the pages that follow, you will find ingenious ways to vary the cabbage soup, dozens of ideas for tastier breakfasts, lunches, and dinners, plus suggestions for using foods in deliciously unexpected ways and at unexpected times of day.

ADD ZING AND VARIETY TO THE SOUP

Even without additional flavoring ingredients, the cabbage soup you will be having every day of the diet is a remarkably good vegetarian soup. It's so good, in fact, that many dieters prefer it as is. Others want more variety, however, and the following ideas offer just that.

Note: You can use these suggestions to season the soup by the batch or by the bowl. Seasoning by the batch—that is, adding flavor ingredients to the soup as it cooks—brings out richer, more developed flavor. Adding the same ingredients in proportionally smaller amounts to the soup after you've ladled it into a bowl gives you the opportunity to sample a variety of combinations over the course of two or three days. Your choice.

The amounts and quantities of flavoring ingredients in the "recipes" that follow are approximations, erring if at all on the side of mildness. If you prefer more robust flavor, just add more.

Cabbage Soup Italiano

- ½ cup chopped flat leaf (Italian) parsley
- 3 to 4 fresh oregano leaves, crushed, or 1 teaspoon dried oregano

Add the ingredients to the soup as it cooks or use smaller amounts of each to flavor one bowl of soup.

Szechuan Cabbage Soup

- 1 to 2 tablespoons soy sauce
- ½ teaspoon Chinese chili paste

Add the ingredients to the soup as it cooks or use smaller amounts of each to flavor one bowl of soup.

Cabbage Soup Deutsch

- 2 teaspoons whole caraway seeds
- 3 sprigs fresh thyme, crushed, or 2 teaspoons dried thyme
- ⅓ cup cider vinegar

Add the ingredients to the soup as it cooks or use smaller amounts of each to flavor one bowl of soup.

Bengal Cabbage Soup

- 2 cucumbers, peeled and sliced
- 2 teaspoons ground cumin
- 2 teaspoons ground turmeric

Add ingredients to the soup as it cooks or use smaller amounts of each to flavor one bowl of soup.

Tex-Mex Cabbage Soup

- 3 to 4 teaspoons chili powder
- 2 jalapeño peppers, finely chopped

Add ingredients to the soup as it cooks or use smaller amounts of each to flavor one bowl of soup.

Cabbage Soup Caribbean

- 1 teaspoon hot sauce
- 1 to 2 teaspoons powdered ginger

Add ingredients to the soup as it cooks or use smaller amounts of each to flavor one bowl of soup.

Sweet and Sour Cabbage Soup

- ⅓ cup cider vinegar
- 1 packet artificial sweetener

Add ingredients to the soup as it cooks or use smaller amounts of each to flavor one bowl of soup.

Savory "Creamed" Cabbage Soup

- ½ cup plain, no-fat yogurt or ½ cup skim milk

Stir yogurt or skim milk into the soup during the last 5 minutes of cooking or stir a smaller amount into one bowl of soup. (Subtract the yogurt or skim milk from your daily allowance.)

WHAT'S FOR BREAKFAST?

Many dieters have had problems with breakfast on the original Cabbage Soup Diet, except on days when unlimited fruit is allowed. Fruit is still the ideal breakfast choice on

Days 1, 3, 4 (bananas only), and 7 of the New Cabbage Soup Diet.

But why stop at a single plain raw fruit? There are lots of other ways to enjoy fruit for breakfast. You can use all the foods on the New Cabbage Soup Diet any way you want to—as long as you don't exceed the suggested amounts (if any), don't add ingredients that contribute extra calories, and don't use foods that are not part of the plan for that day.

Here are a few ideas that will give a scrumptious start to every day of the diet.

Fruit Breakfasts for Free Fruit Days

Fruit Salad
Slice up your choice of fresh fruits, including watermelon and cantaloupe if you have them, and combine in a bowl. Fresh, ripe fruit is usually moist and tempting without adding additional juice, but if you prefer a juicier fruit salad, add a little juice squeezed from a fresh grapefruit or orange. Top it off, if you like, with a sprinkle of cinnamon, nutmeg, or ground cloves. If the fruit is super-tangy, you can sweeten it up by tossing it with some artificial sweetener.

You can't go wrong with any combination of ripe fruit. They're all natural go-togethers. But some of the most delectable fruit salad combinations include:

- Blueberries and peaches
- Oranges, apples, and strawberries
- Pears and plums
- Watermelon, grapes, and kiwi

Fruit Salad Deluxe
To turn fruit salad into fruit salad deluxe, spoon ½ cup plain, no-fat yogurt into a bowl and pile sliced fruit on top. Subtract the amount of yogurt used in the fruit salad from your daily yogurt allowance.

Going Bananas

On Day 4, when you can have as many as six bananas, enjoy at least one of them in the morning, at breakfast. You can have it plain, or you can bake or broil it (see below). Or you can add a sliced banana to ½ cup of plain, no-fat yogurt. (Don't forget to subtract ½ cup of yogurt from your daily yogurt allowance.)

Heavenly Cooked Fruit

Broiled Fruit

High heat from the broiler caramelizes the natural sugars in fruit, and the result is a wonderful "burnt" sugar flavor and aroma that is marvelous to wake up to, especially in winter.

- Broiled grapefruit is a classic. It's as easy as placing ½ grapefruit under the broiler and letting it sizzle until the top begins to brown. Sprinkle on some cinnamon and enjoy.

Other fruits that take to broiling:

- Sliced apples. Slice should be relatively thick, not wafer-thin
- Sliced peaches
- Sliced fresh pineapple
- Bananas sliced in half lengthwise

Do not attempt to broil berries, melons, or any other very juicy fruit, such as very ripe, juicy pears.

Baked Delights

Mention baked fruit, and baked apples come first to mind. But apples aren't the only fruit that take on a wonderfully different, more mellow flavor when cooked in the oven. In fact, almost all fruit can be baked. The exceptions are melons, berries, and other very juicy fruits.

To bake fruit, place it in a 375°F oven. Bake until the fruit softens and begins to bubble. Try using these fruits.

- Banana (on Day 4, the "banana day")
- Peaches
- Plums

When baking peaches or plums, halve the fruit and remove the pit before placing it in the oven.

Great Breakfasts for Nonfruit Days

The bright, tangy flavor of yogurt is a great morning wake-up call, and it's the perfect solution to the problem of what to eat in the A.M. on those days when fruit is not part of the diet.

You may discover that you enjoy the refreshing flavor of plain, no-fat yogurt without adding anything to dress it up. Many people do. (If you don't, you can stir in a little artificial sweetener.) Or you can use the tanginess of plain yogurt as a base and add "top notes" of flavor with other foods. Yogurt is a natural flavor complement to many vegetables, so there are lots of possibilities.

- Mix in fresh, peeled cucumber slices, then sprinkle yogurt with chopped chives.
- Have a yogurt "salad" breakfast on days that allow free vegetables. Just mix in grated raw carrots, beets, and/or slivers of green or red peppers, and any other free vegetables that strike your fancy.
- Potato for breakfast? Why not? On Day 2, when a baked potato is part of the diet, you can quickly microwave a potato, top it with yogurt, and enjoy. Potato in the morning, of course, means no potato later on.

Note: Remember to subtract the yogurt you have at breakfast from your day's allowance.

DELICIOUS MUNCHES FOR LUNCH AND DINNER

Lunches and dinners on the New Cabbage Soup Diet always include a serving of the soup. Have it plain or try one of the variations given earlier in this chapter.

The soup and a perfect piece of luscious ripe fruit (on fruit days) plus your choice of coffee or tea may provide all the lunchtime flavor you will ever want or need. However, there are many alternatives.

Breakfast at Lunch? At Dinner?

Why not? Here's where mix and match comes in. Although the breakfast suggestions mentioned on pages 92 to 94 are perfect ways to start the day, some of them are just as appropriate at midday or in the evening.

Lunch and Dinner Salads

Like fruit for breakfast, salad at lunch or dinner is an obvious choice—and it's an especially good choice on the New Cabbage Soup Diet because the lively flavor and crispness of fresh, raw vegetables, dressed with a little lemon juice, low-cal salad dressing, or yogurt is a wonderful complement to the mellower taste and softer textures of the soup. A simple lettuce and tomato salad is fine, but with the array of free fruits and vegetables to choose from on this diet, you can pack a lot more flavor into your meals.

A "salad" can be just about any combination of vegetables or fruits, so you can really be creative with all the free varieties on the diet days that allow them. A few ideas to get you started:

- Crisp, raw spinach, red onion rings, mushrooms, and sliced tomatoes
- Grapefruit or orange sections (or both) tossed with mixed greens, including various lettuces, watercress, and chopped fresh herbs
- Vegetable slaw, made with grated raw vegetables such as carrots, beets, radishes, frenched green beans, slivered red and yellow peppers and, yes, cabbage

The salad possibilities are unlimited—almost. Use only those free fruits and vegetables listed in chapter 5. Do not use fruit on Days 2, 5, and 6 of the diet. Omit vegetables on Days 1, 4, and 5.

Grilled Vegetables for Lunch or Dinner

You can make a side dish, or an entire meal, out of mixed, grilled vegetables. Grilling brings out a delicious smoky flavor in the vegetables that is very different from the flavor of steamed or boiled. Some of the best vegetables for grilling are:

- Tomatoes, sliced
- Peppers, quartered, with seeds removed
- Large mushrooms
- Thick-sliced onions
- Thick-sliced zucchini

Chicken or Fish for Lunch or Dinner

They're great for lunch or dinner, and on Days 5 and 6, you can have them at both meals. A few ideas:

- ½ grilled chicken breast drizzled with lemon and sprinkled with chopped chives or parsley, plus the soup
- Diced grilled chicken tossed with low-cal salad dressing or a hot sauce/yogurt dressing (yogurt mixed with 1 or 2 drops hot sauce, depending on your heat tolerance), plus the soup
- Broiled fish filet topped with lemon slices, served with a side of grilled tomatoes, plus the soup
- Flaked tuna with yogurt-mustard dressing (4 parts yogurt to 1 part mustard), grilled vegetables, plus the soup

The suggestions in this chapter are just that—suggestions. Try them if you like, or experiment with your own flavor combinations. Just keep the following guidelines in mind:

- Don't use flavoring ingredients that add extra calories.
- With the exception of herbs, spices, vinegars, mustards, hot sauces, and unsweetened fruit spreads, do not use foods that are not part of the diet.
- When you use yogurt as an ingredient or as the basis of a sauce, don't forget to subtract the amount from your daily yogurt allowance.

With these suggestions for flavoring the New Cabbage Soup Diet still fresh in your mind, and with all the other tips and techniques in this book filed away in your brain, it's finally time to take off—pounds, that is.

CHAPTER 10

They Did It, and You Can, Too!:
Seven New Cabbage Soup Diet
Success Stories

Nothing succeeds like success, they say, so let's hear it from seven New Cabbage Soup Dieters—five women and two men—who lost weight with the help of this unique plan. For some it was easy; just eat and lose. Others found they had to meet and overcome problems along the way. Read their stories. Everyone who wants a slimmer, fitter, healthier body can learn from their triumphs.

KAREN, 45, CALIFORNIA

"Just Call Me the Cabbage Soup Poster Girl!"
Karen, a vivacious, dark-haired woman who lives in a small town up the coast from San Francisco, had been thin all her life—until her world came crashing down around her.

"I was always active and busy and just didn't care that much about food," she says. "I was thin and I loved it. At five foot one inch and 90 pounds, they didn't make clothes small enough to fit me, I had to have everything taken in. That was ten years ago," Karen explains.

"Then everything in my life went wrong. The company I worked for cut back on staff and I was let go. At about the same time, the man I was in love with decided to call it quits. It was just too much. I went into a deep depression. I withdrew from my friends, stopped going to the gym."

Karen had always assumed that depressed people lost their appetite and had trouble sleeping. For her, it was just the opposite. "I began to eat and eat and eat," she says. "I spent my days a-weepin' and a-sleepin' and a-eatin'. My whole life was food, bed, and videos. I remember going to the video store for movies and then stopping off at the convenience store and loading up on giant, overstuffed sandwiches and quarts of ice cream. Then I'd hole up in front of the TV and not go out again until I ran out of food."

In five months, Karen says she went from 90 to 125 pounds. When her unemployment insurance ran out, she pulled herself together enough to find a job. As soon as she qualified for health insurance, she went to a therapist, who referred her to a psychiatrist, who prescribed antidepressants.

Therapy and the medication helped Karen climb out of her depression, but even though her mood improved, she continued to sit at home and eat. Two years ago, she tipped the scales at 180 and had developed serious back and knee problems because of the excess weight.

"It became very clear that if I didn't make some changes I'd be an unhappy, unhealthy fat person for the rest of my life."

Karen, like so many people, got most of her diet information from magazines. "All the articles I read about losing weight told me the best way to do it was to eat smaller, well-balanced meals," she says. "I tried so hard. Every Monday morning I'd wake up and vow to eat less. By Tuesday, I'd be famished and obsessing about bread and pasta. And by Wednesday, I'd be back to my old ways and beating myself up because of my lack of self-control."

Karen learned about the New Cabbage Soup Diet from a coworker. "Frankly, I had to laugh when she told me about it. For starters, I don't like cabbage—and whoever heard of a diet that weird, and that strict! But I knew this woman had lost several pounds in one week on the diet, so

I thought, why not? I'll check with my doctor and if she gives me the okay, I'll give it a try."

To her surprise, Karen completed the seven-day cycle without a hitch and lost eleven pounds. Why was she able to stay on the strict New Cabbage Soup Diet for a week when she had had so much trouble simply cutting back on her food intake?

"In a funny way, the strictness and structure of this diet worked to my advantage. It told me exactly what to eat every day. I never had to make a decision about what to eat. I never had to wonder how much of this or how much of that was okay. And I was never hungry because I kept drinking that soup—which I actually began to look forward to. Oh, I won't pretend that I didn't have visions of pizza and macaroni and cheese, but I stuck it out because it was only for seven days. At the end of the week it was like 'Look, Ma, I did it!' I weighed eleven pounds less, and I felt I could conquer the world!"

Unfortunately, Karen slipped back into her old eat-anything-and-everything habits soon after her first seven-day cycle. "It didn't take long to regain the eleven pounds I lost the first time around," she says. "But my eyes were opened to the fact that I *do* have the ability to control my eating. So a few months later I tried the New Cabbage Soup Diet again and lost nine pounds. Once again, I was ecstatic. And that time, instead of lapsing back into my old way of eating, I began to really pay attention to everything I ate. I read up on nutrition. I learned about portion control. I found out how to be more active in spite of my bad back and knees. And now I'm using what I learned to create a better, healthier life."

Karen now weighs 140 pounds. That's still a long way from her goal weight of 110. But she knows she's going to make it. "I credit the success I had with the New Cabbage Soup Diet for giving me the self-confidence I needed to keep going. I guess you could call me the poster girl for that diet!"

BRAD, 29, MICHIGAN

Proud "Guy without a Shirt"

A salesman with an office supply firm outside of Detroit, Brad is single and hopes some day to find "a great gal to spend the rest of my life with." In the meantime, he's having fun, dating lots of young women, going to parties and rock concerts, and hanging out with his friends.

Brad doesn't really have much of a weight problem. In fact, according to the standard height and weight charts, he weighs just about what he should for his height—5 foot 11 inches—and heavy bone structure. He's used to eating whatever he wants whenever he wants it, and usually doesn't give a second thought to his physical appearance. Except in the summer, when he and his friends spend every weekend at a nearby lake.

"A couple of years ago, I started to get this *roll* around my gut. Now, I'm a big guy, but I'm not fat per se, just kind of beefy. And this roll, well, nobody knew it was there but me when I was dressed. I mean, my suits and jeans still fit me, I didn't have to buy a bigger size or anything, it was just there and it bothered me. I'd look at it after showering and think, 'Damn, I've gotta do something about this.' "

But, Brad says, he did nothing, and by the time summer came around again the roll was still there.

"Now, I never thought of myself as one of those guys who care a lot about the way they look. I'm not vain or anything," Brad confides. "But I just felt funny going out to the beach the first time that summer with this *roll*. I remember thinking 'I'm too young to be going to pot, this way.' So I just kept my shirt on. Nobody noticed, nobody said anything, I just sat around on the sand with my shirt on. I'd take it off for a swim, come back, towel off, and put my shirt back on.

"The next winter," Brad continues, "the roll was still there. I was getting used to it, not thinking about it at all anymore, when some of the guys started talking about taking off for a week in the Florida Keys. "Uh-oh. The *roll*. I was up for the trip, but I sure didn't want to spend my beach time in Florida covered up in a shirt."

Brad had a month to do something about the roll. "I quickly joined a gym and started working out. B-o-r-i-n-g, but I did it. A week went by. No difference. Another week. No difference. I stopped drinking beer. I thought I saw a little improvement. Very little. Two weeks left and I swallowed my pride and asked my sister if she knew any diets that would take off a few pounds in a hurry. She told me about a friend of hers who had lost weight on something called the New Cabbage Soup Diet. I laughed. I said, 'You've got to be kidding.' But I bought the book anyway."

According to Brad, making the cabbage soup was the first time in his life he had ever cooked anything more complicated than a scrambled egg. "For me, soup was something that came out of a can, not something you make," he says. "But I followed the recipe and it tasted pretty good."

As for following the diet, Brad had no problems. "I have to say that even though I've always been a meat and potatoes guy, I really enjoyed all those fruits and vegetables. In fact, one of the good things about the diet was that it really got me into vegetables."

But the best thing about the diet, says Brad, is the way it made that roll get smaller. "Don't get me wrong, it didn't go away completely, but it was definitely smaller. And guess what? I got a great tan in Florida 'cause I proudly took my shirt off at the beach!"

Would Brad use the New Cabbage Soup Diet again? "In a minute," he says. "Although I'm still going to the gym and I'm eating better now, so maybe I won't need it. But if I do? It's cabbage soup time!"

JOELLE, 55, CONNECTICUT

"Good-bye Winter Blahs and Bloat"

The mother of three children, all of whom are grown and living on their own, Joelle is an interior designer who lives with her stockbroker husband in a big house with a pool in Connecticut. She's an avid reader and tennis player and volunteers at a homeless shelter.

"I've been slender most of my life," says Joelle. "Even after my pregnancies, the pounds just seemed to melt away. But now that I'm postmenopausal, things are different. I have to be much more careful about what I eat because if I'm not, I gain weight very quickly."

Joelle *is* careful about what she eats, most of the time. She tries to follow the rules of good nutrition with a well-balanced diet that includes lots of vegetables and fruit, whole grains, lean meat, chicken, and fish. Nevertheless, she does put on five or ten pounds every year during the winter months.

"In summer, I'm out there working in the garden and playing tennis or swimming on the weekends, and I walk to and from my office. But like a lot of people, I slow down in the winter. I start to 'hibernate,' spending my evenings reading by the fire or watching TV, going to bed early, that sort of thing. And then, of course, my husband and I are invited to numerous parties during the holidays."

She adds, "Maybe it's because of the lack of exercise, or maybe it's eating all that rich party food, but I also tend to feel sluggish and sort of heavy and blah in the dead of winter.

"And now that I'm older," she continues, "getting rid of that 'winter weight' requires more than just cutting back on certain foods, the way it used to be. It's a real effort and losing those five or ten pounds could take months. That's where the Cabbage Soup Diet comes in."

One January a few years ago, Joelle read about the Cabbage Soup Diet in a magazine. "I looked at the menus and the list of foods and I thought, 'Hmmm, I *like* that, it seems very healthy with all those fruits and vegetables.' Also, I had fond memories of the cabbage soup my mother used to make, so that was something else in its favor. After discussing the diet with my physician, I decided to try it."

If there is anything Joelle prides herself on, it's her discipline. So, getting through the seven-day diet cycle was, as she puts it, "a piece of cake!"

"I enjoyed the meals, and the pounds practically flew off my body. But something else happened that was almost as good. I felt energized after a couple of days on the diet. I felt light and buoyant. I'm not just talking about weighing less, but about actually *feeling* lighter and less bloated and sluggish. It's a wonderful feeling."

Ever since then, Joelle has used the New Cabbage Soup Diet a couple of times each winter. She uses it to lose the pounds she gains as a result of exercising less and eating more—and she uses it to rev up her energy and to get rid of what she calls "winter blahs and bloat."

"I don't know how many other people experience that feeling of lightness and energy when they use this diet," says Joelle. "I just know it works that way for me, and I love it."

SHELLEY, 39, WISCONSIN

"Hugged My Honey and My Tummy Wasn't in the Way!"
"They said it couldn't be done," says blond, blue-eyed Shelley, with a dazzling grin. She's talking about her family, all of them as blond and blue-eyed as she, and all of them big eaters and overweight practically from the day they were born.

"My mother is heavy—oh, let's just say the F word, she's *fat*. So is my father, so is my brother, and so is my sister," Shelley says. "It runs in the family. That's what they say. But you should see what they eat! Huge meals, junk food snacks every hour on the hour.

"Mom was a pretty good cook," Shelley continues.

"Every night the table was piled with platters of chops and bowls of potatoes whipped with butter, and there was always something rich and gooey for dessert. We were one of the few families I knew who actually sat down to dinner together, and we'd all sit around joking and laughing and eating up a storm. Honestly, we were a happy family— make that *fat* and happy family!

"I always had lots of friends, and even though I was overweight I never had trouble attracting men. When I met Dan, my husband, I was at my heaviest—198 pounds and 5 feet 6 inches. He loved me in spite of my size, and I loved him all the more because he accepted me as I was."

Shelley wasn't particularly concerned about her weight until three years ago, when her mother was diagnosed with diabetes and—a few months later—her father had a heart attack. "That was when it hit me, fat can kill! My parents say it's too late for them; they'll stay fat and take the consequences. Well, I hate it that they feel that way, but I'm not going to follow in their footsteps."

After checking with her doctor, Shelley started a long-term weight-loss plan that allowed her to eat moderate amounts of a wide variety of foods.

"It was a perfectly reasonable, healthy diet, but I'm very results-oriented, and I just wasn't getting good results. It took weeks and weeks to lose just a couple of pounds. I felt like I was getting nowhere fast," she says. "If it wasn't for the negative example my parents set, I might have given up."

About six months into her diet, Shelley heard about the New Cabbage Soup Diet. "The idea of alternating between moderate, well-balanced eating with quick weight loss on the Cabbage Soup Diet made so much sense, and my doctor went along with the idea. My first week on Cabbage Soup I lost seven pounds. Compare that to two pounds in a month!"

After that, Shelley's weight-loss routine consisted of three weeks of moderate dieting followed by a week of cabbage soup eating. "It's my no-fail recipe for getting results," she says. "The highlight of it all was one day when I hugged my husband and realized my tummy was no longer in the way!"

Shelley reached her goal weight of 140 pounds six months ago and has been holding steady ever since. "It's not hard because I no longer crave junk food and huge amounts of old favorites like mashed potatoes," she says.

"And if I do gain a pound or so, I take care of it right away with a few days on—you guessed it—the New Cabbage Soup Diet."

LYLE AND MARA, IN THEIR 40s, NEW YORK

"Walking, Water, and Cabbage Soup"

Lyle and Mara have been married twenty years and live with their two school-age children in Staten Island, New York. They share almost everything, including an interest in politics, a desire to make their community a better place, and twenty-five extra pounds each. Now they're even sharing the New Cabbage Soup Diet.

"Neither Mara nor I are obese," Lyle says. "But if we don't start watching it, we could each have a real weight problem in the future. For us, the Cabbage Soup Diet is preemptive. We go on and off at intervals, and we're slowly losing weight and getting fitter."

Mara concurs. "I'm in no big rush to get thin. Although I'm aware of the fact that many people have used this diet to lose pounds in a hurry, what we want to do is slowly get down to a healthier weight and stay there for the rest of our lives."

So one week each month is Cabbage Soup Diet week at their house. Lyle and Mara follow the diet exactly as written. On diet weeks, Mara, who does most of the cooking, prepares a double batch of cabbage soup on Sunday evening so it will be ready to eat when they start the cycle on Monday. Sunday is also the day when they stock up on fresh, frozen, and canned fruits and vegetables, plus yogurt, which they prefer to skim milk.

What about the kids? "Of course, they don't join us on the diet," says Mara, "but on diet weeks, I use the diet plan as a foundation and add foods for the kids. For instance, I'll serve them lots of the free vegetables and fruits Lyle and I are having and augment their meals with meat or chicken or fish, a starch, bread if they want it, and a simple dessert. It's healthy and they're perfectly happy—but I have to admit, they don't care for the soup."

In the year since they started once-a-month New Cabbage Soup Dieting, Lyle is down fourteen pounds and Mara, twelve. Losing weight has inspired other lifestyle changes for the couple. "We're walking several times a week now," Lyle says. "Not just me and Mara, but the kids, too. We're out there pep-walking around the neighborhood after dinner and on the weekends, rain or shine. It's a great family activity and we all enjoy the time together."

"We've also discovered the power of water," Mara chimes in. "I've read that even mild dehydration can affect alertness and energy levels, so we're both drinking at least eight glasses a day now. And you know what? It's working!"

"Walking, water, and cabbage soup . . . are we health nuts, or what?" asks Lyle.

ESTELLE, 31, ILLINOIS

"Out, Out, Damned Clothes!"
Born and bred in a small town in Iowa, Estelle arrived in the Chicago area seven years ago to pursue a career in public relations. She's a friendly, outgoing redhead who speaks with unusual candor about her diet experiences.

"I'll admit it, I used to be obsessed with food and dieting and exercise and being thin. I used to wish sometimes that I'd develop anorexia and get really, really skinny so that I could eat my way back up to normal. How's that for bizarre?"

Throughout her twenties, Estelle's weight seesawed back and forth between a high of 140 and a low of 105 (she is five foot three inches tall), and in the years since college, she had accumulated three wardrobes. She called them her "very fat" clothes, her "fat" clothes, and her "thin" clothes.

"Growing up in Iowa, I was a little bit of a chunk, which was normal for where I lived. It's farm country, and everyone eats these big farm-type meals and nobody bothers much about their weight," says Estelle. "My weight obsession began at college, in Texas, where I quickly gained the 'freshman fifteen.' There were a lot of us chubettes at school—a whole group of us who hung out together, studied together, went to movies together, and we were always stuffing our faces. In the meantime, there were all these other girls, thin girls, with great clothes, and they were dating and going to all the good parties. I envied them, I wanted to be like them. I wanted to get skinny. Skinny as a ballerina, skinny as a fashion model.

"In my career as a dieter," Estelle continues, "I've tried every diet you've ever heard of. I've bought and paid for expensive herbs guaranteed to take off weight. I've tried legal and illegal diet drugs. I've exercised till I thought I'd drop.

"I lost weight dozens of times," Estelle continues. "And I always put it back on again, plus a few extra pounds. It finally registered: It's not that *hard* to lose weight. What's hard is keeping it off. What a revelation! Duh!"

Estelle says she finally "grew up." "I began to accept the fact that I'm not meant to be model-skinny and that I was making myself unhappy trying to be something I'm not. I began to focus on getting down to 115—a good, healthy weight for me—and staying there. The New Cabbage Soup Diet really helps."

On her first seven-day cycle, Estelle lost eight pounds. "That put me within twelve pounds of my goal," she says. "Then I followed the instructions in the book for slow, steady weight loss. When I hit one of those plateaus, where I stopped losing weight for a week or so, I'd go back on the New Cabbage Soup Diet. That's all it took to start losing pounds again! I swear, it's magic!"

Estelle has maintained her weight in the 114- to 116-pound range for a year now. She takes exercise classes three times a week. She has given up soft drinks and high-fat snacks but doesn't obsess about what to eat and what not to eat. And if she gains a couple of pounds? "It's back to cabbage soup!"

Recently Estelle felt sure enough of her ability to keep her weight stable that she went through her closet, removed all her "fat clothes," and took them to a charity thrift store. "It was like out, out damned clothes! I wish everyone with a weight problem could experience that feeling of absolute, utter triumph!"

CHAPTER 11

Day 1

Here and in the next six chapters, you'll find menus and food suggestions for every day of the New Cabbage Soup Diet. Just as important, you will find dozens of ideas and tips—including simple ideas for getting more physical activity into your life—that will make the weight-loss process even easier. Some of the tips are specific to this diet. You can use them over again every time you return to the diet. Others will be equally helpful if and when you decide to switch to a slower, long-term diet—and for controlling your weight throughout the years to come.

Right now, though, before you begin the diet, read through this chapter and the six that follow. They'll provide a useful overview and give you a better idea of what's in store on each day of the diet. They'll also clue you in in advance on how to handle certain challenges—such as cravings, the need for "food soothing," and boredom—should they arise. Then each diet morning, when you awaken, turn to the appropriate chapter for a refresher course.

If you are using the three-day blitz version of the diet, this is Day 1 for you, as well. Use the chapters for Day 1, Day 2, and Day 3. They'll help you look better at the beach, or slim down just enough to fit into favorite clothes that are now too snug.

THE NEW CABBAGE SOUP DIET, DAY 1

On the menu today:

    Cabbage soup
    Unlimited free fruits
    1 8-ounce serving of skim milk, or plain, no-fat
        yogurt
    Tea or coffee, plain, or with artificial sweetener
    Water
    1 tablespoon low- or no-fat salad dressing
    Your choice of herbs, spices, and other low-fat or
        low-cal flavoring ingredients

Reminder: If you start the day with skim milk in your coffee, you are not permitted to switch to yogurt later on in that same day.

WAKE UP AND WEIGH IN

It's a great day to start this diet, so yawn, get up out of bed, and head for the bathroom scale. You'll be weighing yourself just twice on this diet—now, on Day 1, and once again on the morning after you complete Day 7 (or complete Day 3 if you are using the three-day version). To make weighing as accurate as possible, slip out of your robe, urinate, and then step on the scale before going in for breakfast. Record your starting weight in your diet journal.

MEASURE UP

You might want to take measurements, so that you can keep track of the inches you lose. You will certainly want a record of your measurements if you are planning to repeat the New Cabbage Soup Diet in two weeks or more after you finish this first cycle, or if you intend to continue losing weight on a slower, long-term diet.

You'll need a good, flexible plastic tape measure. (Don't

try to use the metal kind; these are fine for measuring walls or windows, but no good at all for measuring the contours of the human body.) In taking measurements, pull the tape tight enough to eliminate slack, but not so tight that it presses into your flesh.

How to take accurate measurements:

- To measure your chest or bust, the tape should snugly encircle your upper back at nipple level.
- To measure your waist, draw the tape snugly around your abdomen at the level of greatest indentation.
- To measure your stomach, draw the tape around your abdomen at belly button level.
- Measure around your hips at their broadest point.
- Measure your thighs about eight inches above the knee (or wherever they are widest).

JOURNAL TIME
In chapter 8, you learned about the importance of keeping a diet journal—not just to record your progress, but to help you stay positive and motivated every step of the way. So right now, before breakfast, take time out to jot a few words of encouragement to yourself. Tell yourself how enthusiastic you are about losing weight on this diet and how you intend to make today a 100 percent success!

BREAKFAST IDEAS
Day 1 is a fruit day. Since there's nothing like the crunch and juicy flavor of fresh ripe fruit for breakfast, have a selection of fruit, as many and as much of each as you want, from the free fruit list. Eat them as is, cut them up and make a fruit salad—or a fruit salad with plain, no-fat yogurt. (See the fruit breakfasts in chapter 9 for more ideas.)

Reminder: If you have yogurt in the morning, you're locked into yogurt for the rest of the day. The diet doesn't allow switching back and forth from yogurt to skim milk. (Of course, you may have skim milk tomorrow, if you want it.)

MINI-WORKOUT

Do some walking today, in the morning, if you can manage it. You don't have to walk very far or for very long, but you *should* walk more than you ordinarily do. A couple of ideas: Walk around the block once or twice before you leave for work, or after you get there. (You don't need workout clothes for this, just comfortable shoes.) If a morning walk is inconvenient, walk in the early evening for ten minutes or so.

Step out with your chest high, shoulders down, and tummy in. Keep the pace brisk yet comfortable. Take long strides and swing your arms.

DAY 1 LUNCH

Cabbage soup, of course, and as many free fruits as you want. This is a good day to have the soup plain, without any flavorful adornments. The soup is new to you now, and you'll enjoy it just as it is. If you didn't pack it in a thermos, be sure to heat it up in the office microwave. Hot soup, remember, is more satisfying and filling than cold.

Reminder: Eat alone if possible. That might mean having a solitary lunch at your desk. If you stay in for lunch, try to go outside for some fresh air when you are finished eating. Window shop, run errands, visit the library if there's one nearby, or just stroll. It's important that lunchtime on the diet gives you the sense that you've had a real break from your work.

MIDDAY SLUMP?

Many people can practically set their clocks by it—that slowed-down, lethargic feeling that occurs at or about three

P.M. each day. That slump is often accompanied by hunger and may be related to lowered blood sugar levels. However, if you had plenty of fruit at lunchtime, and your body is still making use of the natural sugar it contains, you may not experience loss of energy today.

If that slump does occur, have another piece of fruit. (Remember, you can have as much as you want today.) The natural sugar in the fruit should bring your body's blood sugar levels back up again and see you through until dinner. This fruit prescription for midday loss of energy is a good one to use anytime—diet or no diet. The only exception is on nonfruit days of the New Cabbage Soup Diet.

Have the fruit alone, or with a jolt of caffeine. Coffee, as you know, contains more caffeine than tea, so if you are especially prone to caffeine jitters, have tea instead.

PROGRESS CHECK

How are you doing so far? If you're like most people who follow the diet, you're doing just fine, thank you. You might even feel better than usual today—less tired, more peppy, and upbeat. Part of that good feeling certainly has to do with your changed eating pattern, especially if you ordinarily eat richer, fattier foods during the day. Rich foods load you down and can make you feel slow and groggy. Give yourself a figurative pat on the back for starting the diet.

DAY 1 DINNER

Start with hot soup. You may want to try one of the soup flavor variations mentioned in chapter 9. For dessert? You guessed it: fruit. If you're having skim milk instead of yogurt today, you may drink all of it with this meal.

If this is a yogurt day for you, there are several ways to enjoy it at dinner: You can stir some of the yogurt into your soup to make it creamier. You can eat it plain or with the tablespoon of sugar-free fruit spread you are allowed on fruit days. Or you can have yogurt as part of a fruit salad.

HOW TO INCREASE MEALTIME SATISFACTION

You won't feel hungry on the New Cabbage Soup Diet because there's always soup and, on most days, free fruits or vegetables to fill up on. Occasionally you may feel unsatisfied—not because you aren't getting enough to eat, but because your food choices are limited and you can't have all the different foods you might want.

Physical and psychological satisfaction after a meal are extremely important to achieving the results you want on this or any weight-loss program, and there are several proven methods for getting what some people call "more bang for the bite." Put them all together, and satisfaction is almost guaranteed.

Slow Down

Taste, chew, and swallow as slowly and deliberately as possible. It will give your taste buds a chance to fully "register" the flavor and mouth-feel of the food. This is important because complete satisfaction depends almost as much on the *experience* of eating as on having enough to eat.

If you've been a fast eater all your life, you'll have to concentrate on slowing down. Try these techniques:

- Take a sip of water or skim milk between bites of food.
- Place your knife and fork or spoon back on your plate after each bite. Don't pick them up again until you are ready for the next bite.
- Chew your food thoroughly. Don't swallow until it is liquefied.
- If you are eating with your family or housemates, try to be the last one to finish. When you're alone, watch the clock. See if you can stretch your meal out to a full twenty minutes or even a half hour.

Make Meals Special

Attractive food and a properly set table add greatly to the enjoyment of a meal; on the other hand, eating on the run, eating while standing in front of the refrigerator, or eating while you're scanning the paper can feel like no meal at all. Try to make your meals real.

- Don't eat without being seated at a table, with a place mat, plate, napkin, and silverware. These visual cues send a message to your brain that a meal is on the way. You may not have all the amenities when you're eating lunch at the office, but at least clear ample space at your desk, spread a napkin as place mat, and use real utensils instead of plastic.

- Don't combine eating with other activities. No TV, no book, crossword puzzle, or list-making—in short, nothing that comes between you and your food. (Soft, undemanding music, however, the kind you sense rather than actively listen to, is okay, and will probably enhance your enjoyment.) It's important to keep your mind focused on your food. When your attention is elsewhere—and tasting, swallowing, and chewing become reflexive rather than deliberate—it's possible to finish a whole meal without it registering in your brain. You might even leave the table yearning for the meal you've just had!

NONFOOD TREAT TIME!

Back in chapter 6, you were encouraged to reward yourself with a small treat for every day you stay on the diet. Giving yourself a special, pleasurable experience in return for abiding by the rules of the diet can be an effective way to reinforce your commitment and resolve. Now's the time. Whether you choose a long, foamy, luxurious bubble bath or a quick visit to a good friend, don't skip it.

BEDTIME

Today and for the remaining six days of the New Cabbage Soup Diet, you will be urged to write a few lines in your diet journal before turning in for the night. A diet journal, remember, is the place for giving yourself pep talks and pats on the back. (Be sure to date each entry and note which day of the diet you're on; you'll enjoy reading the journal in days to come.) Keep it positive. Congratulate yourself for sticking with the diet throughout the day. Tell yourself how easy it was, as well as how much you enjoyed the walking or other extra activity you engaged in today. Mention the times (if any) that you felt tempted to eat something not on the diet, but resisted the urge. End with enthusiasm for tomorrow—even if you don't feel that way. Getting it down in writing is a way to make the enthusiasm real.

CHAPTER 12

Day 2

Welcome to your second day on the New Cabbage Soup Diet. If you felt marvelous yesterday, before you went to bed, you're probably feeling even better this morning: lighter, more energetic, full of confidence, eager to start the day and meet head-on every diet challenge that comes your way.

Some dieters, in fact, do find Day 2 the most challenging day on the diet because where food is concerned, this is the most restrictive day. Be sure to read this chapter through right now. That way, you'll be ready for all the diet-related challenges you might have to face.

Let's take a look at what you'll be eating in the next twenty-four hours:

THE NEW CABBAGE SOUP DIET, DAY 2

On the menu today:

    Cabbage soup

    Unlimited free vegetables

    1 large baked potato

    1 8-ounce serving skim milk, or plain, no-fat yogurt
        (You may have plain, no-fat yogurt on your po-
        tato if you like. *Remember:* If you choose this
        option, you must not have skim milk today.)

Tea or coffee, plain, or with artificial sweetener
Water
1 tablespoon low- or no-fat salad dressing
Your choice of herbs, spices, and other low-fat or
  low-cal flavoring ingredients

WAKE-UP CALL

Don't weigh yourself this morning. Do spend a few minutes
with your diet journal telling yourself how good it feels
to—finally—be doing something about the pounds you
want to lose. You learned in chapter 6 how important it is
to approach any major endeavor one step at a time, so think
of today as your second giant step to a healthier, slimmer
body.

BREAKFAST IDEAS

Fruit is the obvious breakfast food of choice whenever it
is allowed on the diet. Today, however, is not a fruit day,
so it's yogurt to the rescue. If you like the tangy, refreshing
flavor of plain yogurt, here's the perfect opportunity to enjoy it. Otherwise, try flavoring your yogurt with one of the
yogurt-plus-vegetables breakfast suggestions in chapter 9.
If you want to use yogurt as a sour-cream substitute for the
potato you'll be eating later on today, make sure to save
enough. If yogurt alone leaves you feeling less than satisfied and you want more food, heat up a bowl of cabbage
soup. You'll be surprised at how satisfying it can be in the
morning.

MINI-WORKOUT

Before you get into the shower, do a minute or so of jogging in place to burn off a few extra calories and to rev
you up for the rest of the day. Music can help you get into
the swing, so turn on the radio and hunt around until you
find something upbeat with an easy rhythm, or slip an up-

beat CD into your CD player. As you jog, keep your knees
flexed (you want a loose, bouncing motion), bend your elbows, and pump your arms.

ELEVEN O'CLOCK STRETCH
Many people need a short break at about this time in the
morning. Stretching is ideal. It's pleasurable, relieves stress,
and takes just a few minutes. Try this:

Stand tall (if convenient, take your shoes off) and reach
for the ceiling with your arms and hands. You want that
stretch to "open" the middle section of your body as it lifts
your chest up and away from your abdomen. Try yawning.
Somehow it adds to the enjoyment of a good, long stretch.
How long you hold the stretch is up to you, but really try
to get into it.

Now, if you have time, try one or both of these stretch
variations.

- Stretch as above, but instead of standing flatfooted,
  go up on your toes and *really* reach for the ceiling.
- In the basic stretch position (arms lifted high, mid-
  section open), shift your weight from one foot to the
  other. You'll feel a pleasant, alternating pull from
  your armpits down to your hips with each weight
  change.

DAY 2 LUNCH
Today you will have a bowl of hot cabbage soup and veggies, veggies, veggies. Some of you might want to have the
baked potato you're allowed on Day 2 at lunchtime. Go
ahead if that's your preference. Food choices on the New
Cabbage Soup Diet are restricted, but there are no rules
governing the time and the order in which you eat the various foods you are allowed.

AFTERNOON PICKUP—THE "EHHH . . . WHAT'S UP, DOC?" SOLUTION

Don't even bother with this section if you're feeling great and functioning in top form today. But if, like so many other people—on a diet or not—your energy level takes a dip some time in the middle of the afternoon, you may want something to eat now.

Fruit would be the best choice because of the natural sugar it contains, but this is not a fruit day. However, vegetables with a high sugar content are almost as good. Chief among the higher-sugar veggies you are allowed on this diet are carrots, so why not use them to pick you up if you're feeling down? You can have as much as you want of raw, steamed, or canned carrots. Or you can have carrot juice—an even better choice because the natural sugar content is somewhat higher.

Higher-sugar raw, steamed, or canned vegetables such as beets and parsnips are other options.

Have tea or coffee with your vegetable pickup if you want it. The caffeine in either can help boost alertness and energy levels in the middle of the day. *Remember:* You can have as much tea or coffee as you want on the New Cabbage Soup Diet, but a word of caution is in order. Consume these caffeine-containing beverages in moderation. The diet is so low in calories and fat that the caffeine in tea or coffee might have a greater effect on your body than it would otherwise, and increased feelings of tenseness and stress may result. That's just what you *don't* want now.

DAY 2 DINNER—FLAVOR IT UP

Dinner is soup, free vegetables with your choice of low-fat, low-cal salad dressing or other flavorings, plus that potato if you haven't already eaten it at lunchtime. You also can have coffee or tea. If you decide not to finish your skim milk or plain, no-fat yogurt now, be sure to have it before you go to bed.

Important: Why You Should Add Extra Flavor on Day 2
Remember that some cabbage soup dieters have found Day 2 to be more challenging than any other day on the diet. Day 2, after all, is the strictest day, with the narrowest range of flavors. Although you won't feel real hunger because you can have all the veggies and cabbage soup you want, your taste buds, your mouth, and your brain may not register full satisfaction with this narrower range of flavors. Since a variety of interesting and pleasing flavors helps keep your mouth happy and your brain satisfied, this is a day to use plenty of flavoring ingredients in the soup and vegetables. Why not skip back to chapter 9 and take another look at the soup and vegetable flavor variations it contains.

NONFOOD TREAT TIME!
Sometime this evening, do something that you really enjoy. Anything at all is okay—except eating a favorite food. Back in chapter 6 you learned why: Giving yourself a small treat at the end of each successful diet day helps you stay motivated and committed. As you progress through each of the next few days, you'll find yourself looking forward to the evening and the pleasurable activity you'll engage in then. And that spark of anticipation might help see you through any rough moments you might encounter on the diet.

There's another reason to give yourself a nonfood after-dinner treat, and that is to minimize feelings of deprivation. Psychological studies suggest that dieters who feel deprived and say to themselves "It's not fair that I have to eat less than everyone else in the family," or "Poor me, all the things I enjoy are forbidden" are less successful than those who come to terms with the fact that eating less of certain foods is a must if they are going to change their bodies and their lives. Your treat, then, is not just a reward; it's also a tool to help you avoid thoughts and feelings that can damage your chances for success.

GREAT DAY, GOOD NIGHT

Just before you turn in, get out your diet journal and jot down a few compliments to yourself. You've earned the accolades. After all, you've just come through the most difficult day on the New Cabbage Soup Diet—and you did it with flying colors!

CHAPTER 13

Day 3

You're really feeling terrific today, not least because you navigated through Day 2, the most restrictive day on the New Cabbage Soup Diet, the day that so many dieters before you have found to be the most challenging one. You deserve every figurative pat on the back you give yourself. Nothing succeeds like success, and you've proven to yourself that you've got what it takes to achieve your goal.

You should be pleased with yourself even if Day 2 was in fact very easy for you. Knowing that you were able to do easily what others find difficult tells you how committed you are. And as you know, commitment and motivation are the keys to good results in weight loss—as well as to success in any endeavor you put your mind to.

Day 3, because it offers you more in the way of flavor and variety, should be a breeze. *Reminder:* Read this chapter before you start the day so you'll be able to plan ahead in terms of food, treats, and the activities that will help you burn off extra calories.

THE NEW CABBAGE SOUP DIET, DAY 3

On the menu today:
    Cabbage soup
    Unlimited free vegetables

Unlimited free fruit
1 8-ounce serving of skim milk, or plain, no-fat
     yogurt
Tea or coffee, plain, or with artificial sweetener
Water
1 tablespoon low- or no-fat salad dressing
Your choice of herbs, spices, and other low-cal or
     no-cal flavoring ingredients
(No baked potato today)

RISE AND SHINE

Don't weigh yourself.

Get out your journal and record in black and white your positive feelings about yesterday, as well as how well you intend to do today. Tell yourself how proud you are, how strong and confident you feel, and how eager you are to get on with Day 3. Positive self-talk, remember, is one of your most important tools in successful weight loss. The principles of positive self-talk apply just as much to the words and phrases you write in a journal as they do to the words and phrases you use in thinking or talking about yourself. So lay it on thick!

There will certainly be times on the diet when you *don't* feel 100 percent confident and when you *won't* believe—at first—the good things you write about yourself in your journal. It doesn't matter. What matters is that you form positive words and phrases in your mind, and transfer them to paper. When you do that, amazing things happen. Your mind wraps itself around the words, the words begin to shape your feelings, your feelings start to change in ways that reflect the mood and meaning of your self-talk.

BREAKFAST

You can choose from the entire range of free fruits and vegetables for breakfast on Day 3, and you can have as many of them as you want. You can add plain, no-fat yogurt to the fruit if you want to. And all the flavoring ideas in chapter 9 are permitted. So enjoy.

Reminder: If you have yogurt at breakfast, you are not allowed to switch to skim milk later in the day.

MINI-WORKOUT

Some form of easy morning activity is important, so don't skip it. It will help burn off a few extra calories as it clears your head, warms your muscles, and sets you up for the day.

If the weather is fine, take a brisk walk around the block once or twice before you head off to work. Or plan to arrive at work a few minutes early so that you can do some walking before you get down to business. See if you can walk a little farther and a little more briskly than you did on Day 1.

If it's raining, do some jogging in place. If you were able to jog in place for a full minute yesterday, aim for ninety seconds today.

Whatever you choose to do, stop immediately if you begin to feel dizzy, have trouble catching your breath, or your body begins to protest in any other way. These symptoms are not unusual in people who are very overweight or unaccustomed to any exercise at all.

Reminder: The mini-workout suggestions are no more than suggestions. Don't feel you have to comply with them fully or limit yourself to the ones in this book. The idea is not for you to carry out these specific suggestions, but to do whatever you can to get a little more activity into your life.

Note: If you can manage a second round of activity at your office or workplace, or later on at home, so much the better.

DAY 3 LUNCH

As on every New Cabbage Soup Diet day, lunch should include a bowl of hot cabbage soup. If you haven't yet experimented with the flavor variations given in chapter 9, now is a good time to do so. The Italian version of the soup is especially tasty and so is the one called Cabbage Soup Deutsch. (Cabbage and caraway seeds were practically made for each other.) You'll be surprised at how different—and delicious!—the soup can be when you add a few no- or very low-cal seasonings.

Have veggies raw or cooked just until they are slightly softened. Finish lunch with a fruit dessert.

Reminder: Whenever possible, avoid business lunches that require you to have your meal at a restaurant. On days when you have no choice, order a fruit salad (on fruit days) or a leafy green salad (on vegetable days). Be sure to specify no dressing or low-cal, low-fat dressing.

MENTIONING THE UNMENTIONABLE

Sometimes, in some people, the vegetables and fruits on the diet produce flatulence—gassiness in other words. Some of the most notorious of these gas-producing foods are beans, cauliflower, and—yes—cabbage.

Fiber is the culprit here. The problem seems to occur mainly when we consume the kind of fiber that is often called soluble, or digestible fiber. (Insoluble fiber tends to pass through the body without causing this annoying condition.) Soluble fiber is a component of the above-mentioned foods, and of many others as well. When these and other foods that are high in soluble fiber enter the large intestine, they are set upon by the billions of bacteria that make their home there. When the resident bacteria go to work, a few nutrients are freed up (most nutrients are absorbed earlier, in the stomach and small intestine), and waste products are produced. A by-product of all this activity is gas, with or without bloating or abdominal discomfort.

It's very possible that you will complete your seven- or three-day cycle of the diet with no gassy symptoms at all.

If you are afflicted, however, there are ways to minimize
and even prevent the problem.

How to Prevent Gas . . . and Deal with It When It Occurs

- Get a head start on digestion by thoroughly chewing
  all your food. This will help break down fiber in the
  vegetables and fruit even before it hits your stomach.
  The more completely broken down digestible fiber is
  when it reaches your large intestine, the less likely
  you are to have trouble with it.
- Use a product such as Beano, a noncaloric liquid containing food enzymes that make fiber more digestible.
  These products are available at health food stores and
  many drugstores and supermarkets. Package directions instruct you to add a few drops of the product
  to the first bite of food. Don't add Beano or similar
  products to food as it cooks, since heat can deactivate
  the enzymes.
- Don't drink carbonated water with your meals. Car-
  bonation produces air bubbles in the water, and swallowing air can contribute to the discomfort associated
  with gas.
- If you begin to experience a gas attack, try an over-
  the-counter product that helps combat indigestion.

BREAK TIME

Treat midafternoon lassitude, if it occurs, with another serving of cabbage soup or a fruit snack. If you choose fruit,
select one of the sweeter free varieties listed in chapter 5.
An orange, ripe peach, or plum would be ideal. Keep in
mind that fruit that is not yet fully ripened contains less
sugar and may provide less of the mood lift and energy
boost you want now. You may have tea or coffee with your
fruit.

If you can leave the building for a few minutes, take a
quick walk around the block. It can do wonders to clear

your head and refocus your mind. If you must stay indoors, try some long, lazy stretches, as described in chapter 12.

DAY 3 DINNER

Have as much soup and as many free fruits and vegetables as you want. Day 3 dinner can be a veritable banquet because you are allowed unlimited amounts of all these foods.

For a real taste treat, try grilling an assortment of vegetables, including mushrooms. Grilling brings out a slightly different taste and aroma, while the mushrooms contribute an almost meaty texture to the mix. Be sure to slice vegetables destined for the grill into same-size pieces so they'll cook at approximately the same rate.

NONFOOD TREAT TIME!

Once again it's time to reward yourself and reinforce your resolve with a small but special treat. If you indulged in the same treat on Day 1 and Day 2, why not try something different this evening? The variety alone will help keep you happy and motivated.

The treat should be a top priority—more important than finishing household chores, paying bills, or any of the minutiae of daily life that can get in the way of pure enjoyment. You need that treat, you deserve it, and except in cases of emergency, you should make the time for it.

AND SO TO BED . . .

Even if you can hardly keep your eyes open, don't turn out the light until you write a few lines in your journal. Congratulate yourself on a splendid Day 3, and make Day 4 even better by planting strong, confident thoughts in your mind right now, before you go to sleep.

Special congratulations if you're on the three-day version of the New Cabbage Soup Diet. You did it! And when you step on the bathroom scale tomorrow morning, you'll

get your reward: more pounds lost than you ever thought
possible in less than half a week! For even more gratifying
results, you can, of course, continue with the diet. If you
decide to stop tomorrow, wait at least two weeks before
you start a second three-day cycle.

CHAPTER 14

Day 4

In some offices, Wednesday is called "hump day" because it falls in the middle of the work week, and it's all downhill until Friday. No matter what day of the week you started the New Cabbage Soup Diet, Day 4 is "hump day." It's the middle day of the seven-day cycle, and it gets easier, and more interesting, from here on in.

After three days on the diet, your confidence should be sky high. You know you can handle the strictness and structure of the diet, and you feel good about the discipline and will to succeed you've discovered in yourself. Let these good feelings buoy you up and carry you on.

As for why the diet is characterized as being more interesting from now on, one look at the Day 4 menu—as well as those for tomorrow and the next day—will clue you in.

Reminder: Be sure to skim through this chapter first thing today so that you'll know in advance what's in store for you where food, activities, and special challenges are concerned.

THE NEW CABBAGE SOUP DIET, DAY 4

On the menu today:
     Unlimited cabbage soup
     3 to 6 bananas

8 8-ounce servings of skim milk, or 7 8-ounce
    servings of skim milk and 1 8-ounce serving
    of plain, no-fat yogurt
Tea or coffee, plain or with artificial sweetener
Water
Your choice of herbs, spices, and other low-cal or
    no-cal flavoring ingredients (This applies
    every day that you are on the diet.)

All those bananas certainly are a dramatic departure
from the foods you've been eating in the past three days.
This shift in emphasis comes at just the right time. You've
probably been eating more ripe fresh fruits and lightly
cooked vegetables than you ever have before. But as delectable and healthful as they are, your brain and your taste
buds may be crying our for something different now.
You're getting bored, in other words. Today will fix that.

UP AND AT IT

Pull out your diet journal, give yourself full credit for coming this far, tell yourself how committed you are to going
the distance. Emphasize the idea that today's diet is different and that you are really looking forward to getting on
with it.

BREAKFAST!

Bananas. Have one or two plain, broiled, or sliced into yogurt or skim milk. Some dieters like to mix a *mashed* banana with skim milk. They find that the resulting rich,
smooth, thick—and sweet—puree is a welcome change of
pace from the crisp textures of the vegetables they've been
eating.

You must consume seven 8-ounce glasses of skim milk
today (eight, if you're not planning to have yogurt), so be
sure to include a glass at breakfast.

MINI-WORKOUT

If you've enjoyed the short morning walks you've been taking, keep it up. Just try to walk a little farther and longer today and in the days that follow. You may need to set the alarm to go off a little earlier so that you have enough time to walk before you start the working part of your day—a horrendous suggestion if you are one of those who prefer to sleep as late as possible. Try to look at it this way: Hard as it may be to get out of bed earlier, once you're up and around, those few minutes of lost sleep will be forgotten. And the feelings of satisfaction that result from doing something good for yourself—and important to the success of your diet—will make this small sacrifice well worth it.

If you prefer to stay indoors, do some more jogging in place today. Go for at least fifteen seconds more than you did last time.

Skipping or jumping rope in place are other, somewhat more strenuous options. Try them if you feel up to it.

Whatever exercise you choose for starting the day, see if you can arrange to repeat the activity later in the day, either at work or when you are back home in the evening.

Reminder: Shortness of breath, feelings of dizziness, and any muscular or other discomfort are important signals from your body telling you to stop immediately.

DAY 4 LUNCH

Start with a bowl of hot cabbage soup, then have one or two bananas. It's not easy carrying cooked bananas from home, so if today is a workday, your best bet is to bring raw bananas and peel and eat them at lunchtime. Take a few moments to really savor their smooth texture and unique flavor. Bananas really *are* different from the other foods you've been having on the diet, so give your taste buds and brain plenty of time to register the difference. Finish with one or two 8-ounce glasses of skim milk.

Note: You'll be happy to know that bananas are much

easier to digest than the vegetables and fruits called for by the diet up until now: Many babies are introduced to solid foods in the form of mashed bananas because they're so digestible. For the same reason, the very old and the very ailing usually are able to tolerate bananas better than other solid foods. (In fact, it has been said of bananas that they're the first and last real food a person ever gets.) What does this greater digestibility mean for you? Simply that eating easy-to-digest bananas should eliminate much of the gassiness—caused by the abundance of foods containing harder-to-digest fiber—that may have bothered you yesterday and the day before.

THREE P.M. AND ALL'S WELL

The sugars in your lunchtime bananas probably will keep you feeling awake and alert for the rest of the afternoon. However, everyone is different in terms of constitution as well as energy demands and output, so if your spirits and vitality start to wane, have a bowl of hot cabbage soup, a banana, a glass of skim milk, or all three to perk you up in the middle of the day.

Note: Skim milk is most refreshing and satisfying when drunk icy cold. If you brought yours from home and haven't refrigerated it, you can make it more enjoyable simply by adding an ice cube. Try it if your office is equipped with a mini-fridge with ice tray.

Reminder: Caffeine, of course, can be invaluable as a midafternoon pickup. (People don't go on coffee or tea breaks at this time of day for nothing.) But don't have a caffeinated beverage if it makes you feel jumpy or on edge.

Stretching, jogging in place, or a quick walk around the block will provide an additional energy boost now.

WHAT ABOUT FOOD CRAVINGS?

It has been said many times in this book that you will never feel hungry on the New Cabbage Soup Diet because you always can fill up on the soup or on free vegetables or fruits when they are allowed. These foods are enough to keep most dieters feeling full and satisfied. But a few others feel hungry no matter how much cabbage soup or free vegetables or fruits they consume. You may be one of those others.

But is it really hunger? Probably not. More likely, what you are experiencing when you eat your fill of foods allowed on the diet but still do not feel satisfied is a *craving* for food. Hunger is what happens when your stomach is empty and sends out signals calling for more food. Hunger in extreme cases can be painful. Most Americans are fortunate in never having felt true hunger.

Food cravings sometimes are linked to boredom or dissatisfaction. Often we crave something different to eat because we're tired of the same old thing. Other times we feel like eating something because there's nothing else to do, or because what we're supposed to be doing doesn't engage our interest or attention. In those instances, what we really want when we say we are "hungry," or crave food, is diversion—something to entertain ourselves with. If you think about your "hunger" and decide it might actually be a symptom of boredom, change what you have been doing. Invent a different activity if possible. When the time and the place make it imperative to continue your present activity, at least recognize the "hunger" for what it is—a craving. Knowing that dissatisfaction is probably a desire for diversion rather than food redefines it and helps you shift your focus from wanting to eat to wanting to find a more interesting use of your time.

True food cravings do exist, of course. Cravings for high-fat, high-calorie, and high-carbohydrate foods are well documented. These cravings often are described as the brain's demand for nutrients from which it can make more serotonin, a natural chemical that helps ease feelings of stress and tension. Often a small amount of a high-carbohydrate food provides the "cure" for these cravings. A banana is high in carbs and can be useful in curbing cravings today. Cravings on other New Cabbage Soup Diet days may be harder to handle with food. High-sugar fruits can help, so reach for one on free fruit days. As for days when fruit is not a part of the diet, try managing your cravings as you would if they were generated by boredom: by finding something more interesting to do. Learning and using this technique has helped many dieters achieve success.

DAY 4 DINNER

As always, cabbage soup is the entrée tonight. Fill up on it, then have a "dessert" of as many bananas as it takes to fulfill the Day 4 requirement. Dress them up, if you feel like it, with one of the ideas for adding more flavor to bananas in chapter 9. Unless you want to save it for bedtime, drink the remainder of your skim milk requirement.

Reminder: Check your cabbage soup supply. If you're running low, make another batch this evening.

NONFOOD TREAT TIME!

Don't skip your treat even if today, with its infusion of new tastes and textures, hardly felt like dieting at all. Abiding by the rules of the diet, and being rewarded for doing so, helps keep you on track and fully motivated. For this evening, how about something that's not just fun, but a little outrageous or at least out of the ordinary? Something you wouldn't think of otherwise, such as bowling, roller skating, ice skating, bike riding, a few rounds of charades, twenty questions, Trivial Pursuit . . . you get the idea.

SLEEP TIME

Before drifting off, write a few lines in your diet journal. Tell yourself how easy it was today and how great it feels to take control of your food and your life. Then jot down a few confidence-building thoughts to sleep on.

CHAPTER 15

Day 5

You're more than halfway through your first seven-day cycle of the New Cabbage Soup Diet now, and your confidence and motivation have been building since Day 1. The following three days (counting today) should be easier than the first part of the diet for several reasons: You've established a routine and have an idea of what you can expect from the diet, your body, and your mind as you go through each day. You're taking control of your weight and your life, and it feels good—so good you don't ever want to lapse into your old, undisciplined way of eating and living. And the menus for the next two days offer you a range of interesting flavors and textures that have been absent from the diet until now.

If you are like so many others who have followed the New Cabbage Soup Diet, you're really ready for today's big food change. Just as yesterday's bananas may have given you the feeling that you weren't on a diet at all, the chicken and/or fish you will be having today also might make you forget that you are eating to lose weight. But that's exactly what you are doing. The weight-loss process is on track and proceeding full speed ahead.

Reminder: Read this chapter through before you begin the day. It will help you plan for the twenty-four hours to come, answer questions that might arise, and give you a handful of tips to make Day 5 even easier.

THE NEW CABBAGE SOUP DIET, DAY 5

On the menu today:
Unlimited cabbage soup
Unlimited fish or chicken
1 28-ounce can of tomatoes, whole or crushed, or
   up to 6 fresh, ripe tomatoes
1 8-ounce serving skim milk or plain, no-fat yogurt
Tea or coffee, plain or with artificial sweetener
Water
1 tablespoon low- or no-fat salad dressing
Your choice of herbs, spices, and other low-cal, low-
   fat flavoring ingredients

In chapter 5, it was suggested that you choose the lowest-fat chicken and the leanest varieties of fish. Those guidelines are repeated here for your convenience:

Chicken
- Leanest: smaller broiling and frying chickens
- Next best: chicken for roasting
- Avoid: hens and capons

Fish
- Leanest: white-fleshed fish, such as halibut, haddock, flounder, cod, and scrod
- Next best: tuna, bluefish, catfish. (You may have one large serving of any of these today, in addition to leaner varieties. If you want to use canned tuna, choose the solid-pack white variety packed in water.)
- Avoid: darker-fleshed fish like swordfish, mackerel, salmon.

Note: If this is a workday for you, be sure to pack enough chicken or fish to see you through lunch and still have enough left over for a quick afternoon pickup.

GOOD MORNING!

Don't gear up for the day without writing in your diet journal: Give yourself more pats on the back. Make confident statements like "Nothing can stop me now." Tell yourself how great it feels to be in control of your eating and your life.

BREAKFAST!

Today is not a fruit day, but who says the best days on the New Cabbage Soup Diet always begin with fruit? Fish for breakfast is a tradition in some countries, so why not have a broiled or grilled fish fillet—just as if you were breakfasting in an English country house or out camping in the wild! Serve it with plenty of lemon juice to bring up the flavor. Another option: canned solid-pack white tuna, also with lemon juice. If you'd rather have a fishless breakfast, choose plain, no-fat yogurt. (See chapter 9 for flavoring ideas.)

Reminder: If you start the day with yogurt, you are not permitted to switch to skim milk later on.

MINI-WORKOUT

Are you ready to add something new to your repertoire of morning activity? Try a little "weight lifting." You won't need real weights, just a straight-back chair and a couple of hardcover books weighing between one and two pounds each. Here are two easy exercises to get you started.

1. Sit in a chair with your chest lifted, your back straight and slightly away from the back of the chair, and a book balanced on the palm of each hand. Slowly raise and straighten your arms until they are fully extended to each side at shoulder level. Bounce your arms (gently; you don't want to bounce the books off your palms), or simply hold in place for thirty seconds or as long as you can.

2. Still seated in the chair with your chest lifted and your back slightly away from the chair back, grasp a book in each hand. Bend and lift your elbows, keeping your arms close to your ears. (Your hands, still grasping the books, should be positioned behind and close to the base of your neck.) Slowly raise your hands until your arms are straight and reaching toward the ceiling. Hold for five seconds, then slowly bend your arms until your hands are close to the base of your neck again. Repeat five times. Try for more if you can.

Finish your mini-workout with some jogging in place.

DAY 5 LUNCH

Lunch today is practically a feast. Start with a serving of hot cabbage soup. Go on to as much as you like of grilled, broiled, or roasted chicken or grilled or broiled fish. Add a large portion of sliced tomatoes.

If you've been wanting to have lunch at a restaurant, you can safely do so today or tomorrow. Just be sure to choose a place with plain broiled or grilled fish or chicken on the menu.

Eating with other people, remember, can be risky, which is why you were urged in chapter 8 to eat alone as often as your circumstances allow. In addition to the reasons given there, there's still another rationale for eating alone: Dieters and nondieters alike tend to eat more in social situations; they are especially likely to consume more food than they planned to when they eat with friends, coworkers, or other people whom they know well. One study, conducted by researchers at the University of Toronto, found that women volunteers (believing that they were participating in research on responses to the media—a "catch a movie and grab something to eat" scenario) ate an average of 700 calories' worth of food. That was twice as much as what the control group of solitary eaters consumed. Forewarned is forearmed.

Reminder: No vegetables and fruits other than tomatoes today.

QUICK AFTERNOON PICKUPS

It's very possible that you won't need food to perk you up this afternoon. That's because, if you have been following the meal suggestions for Day 5, your body has been supplied with an abundance of protein. What does protein have to do with it? Just this: Because of its composition and the way your body digests it, protein helps maintain steady blood sugar (glucose) levels. When blood sugar levels remain steady, you are far less likely to experience some of the symptoms associated with low blood sugar, including lassitude, fatigue, and crankiness.

But what if you need a quick pickup anyway? Have a cup of tea or coffee. The caffeine should provide an almost-instant energy boost. You can also have more chicken or fish. They won't give you the same quick lift you'd get with sweet, ripe fruit or high-sugar vegetables, but the slower-acting protein in the chicken or fish will tide you over and keep you feeling alert for hours.

Reminder: Stretching, jogging in place, or a quick walk are terrific energizers.

DAY 5 DINNER

Start with a serving of hot cabbage soup. Move on to more broiled or grilled chicken or fish. Have sliced tomatoes on the side or use them to make a sauce. It's easy. Just puree the tomatoes in a blender or force them through a sieve, add lemon juice, garlic, or dill, and your choice of other seasonings. Warm in a saucepan, and pour over the chicken or fish.

Unless you want to have it at bedtime, finish your skim milk or yogurt.

No dessert today. None of the foods permitted on Day 5 are sweet enough. But with all that high-protein food, you certainly won't miss it.

NONFOOD TREAT TIME!

Remember, a small nonfood indulgence each day helps keep you from feeling deprived and unhappy. Plus, it's part of the promise you made to yourself when you started the New Cabbage Soup Diet. Keep it up.

Go back to one of the activities you enjoyed on previous diet days, or think up something new and pleasurable. If you're short on ideas, flip back to chapter 6, where you'll find a number of suggestions.

LIGHTS OUT

As always, spend a few moments writing in your diet journal before you turn in for the night. Now is the time to flood your mind with good thoughts about yourself and the progress you are making. In a sense, those thoughts become "concrete" when you put them down on paper. You also might enjoy reading some of your earlier entries. All of that positive self-talk will percolate in your mind and really set you up for Day 6.

CHAPTER 16

Day 6

By now, you're an expert at following the diet. Your outlook is great, and you are filled with energy—maybe even bubbling over with it. You're feeling lighter, there's a spring to your step, and you're ready for whatever Day 6 may bring. And it's all because you're learning how to manage your food intake and assume responsibility for your weight, and your life. You're on a real losing streak, so keep it going.

Where food is concerned, today, like yesterday, is one of the less demanding days on the diet. There's lots to eat, including plenty of animal protein, which takes your body longer to digest and, like fiber, helps keep you feeling satisfied. Actually, today is even better than yesterday because you can have your fill of free vegetables as well.

Reminder: Read this chapter from beginning to end so that you can plan meals ahead of time and, if necessary, shop for foods you don't have in your kitchen now. It also will give you some problem-solving techniques to help you through difficult moments, should they arise.

THE NEW CABBAGE SOUP DIET, DAY 6

On the menu today:
    Unlimited cabbage soup
    Unlimited broiled or grilled chicken and fish

Unlimited free vegetables
1 8-ounce serving skim milk, or plain, no-fat yogurt
Tea or coffee, plain or with artificial sweetener
Water
Your choice of herbs, spices, and other low-cal or
no-cal flavoring ingredients

Note: Be sure that some of the vegetables you eat today are leafy greens. There's quite a range from which to choose, including spinach, kale, mustard and collard greens, chicory, endive, and lettuces in all their endless variety.

WAKE UP WITH A SMILE!
It's a great day to be alive and a great day to continue with the diet that is helping you lose more pounds and inches than you ever thought possible in just a week. Don't yield to the temptation of weighing yourself. Counting today, you still have two days to go. Instead, do what you've been doing every morning of the diet, write some positive thoughts in your diet journal. Tell yourself how marvelous you feel and how you know beyond a doubt that you are going to make this another successful day.

BREAKFAST!
Think in terms of a savory breakfast featuring fish. Really flavor it up with your choice of fresh herbs such as dill, chives, or basil. For a nice touch, add some sliced or chopped onions. (You may add the onions to the fish as it broils or grills; to prevent burning, wait until the fish is cooked halfway before you sprinkle them on.) Just before eating, add the bright, tangy flavor of lemon juice.)

Plain yogurt is always a breakfast option, so have it instead of the fish if you prefer.

Reminder: If you start out with yogurt for breakfast, you are not permitted to switch to skim milk later in the day.

MINI-WORKOUT

Walk, jog in place, or repeat the easy exercises with weights you learned about yesterday. Whichever activity you choose, see if you can do it a little longer than you have in the past.

DOING THINGS THE HARD WAY

Today is also a good day to start burning off a few extra calories by doing ordinary things the hard way. The idea might seem counterproductive. After all, getting things done quickly with the least expenditure of energy is the goal in most areas of human endeavor. But it's different with weight loss.

Anything you can do to increase your level of physical activity will help you lose more weight more quickly on this diet or off. Anything. Walking down the hall to talk to a coworker uses more energy—which is another way of saying it burns off more calories—than phoning or e-mailing. Standing up and reaching for a file placed high on a shelf uses more energy than pulling the file out of a desk drawer. Anything that can be done "by hand" instead of mechanically—from mowing the lawn to sharpening a knife—will accelerate the weight-loss process. Of course, individually none of these small exertions will burn off more than just a few extra calories. But the accumulated effort over a period of days can make a real difference. Starting today, and continuing for as long as you want to lose weight or maintain your weight loss, try to get into the habit of doing things the hard way. In addition to the few examples given above, you can:

- Walk or bicycle to the store instead of driving or sending someone else.
- Rake leaves and pull weeds instead of having your spouse or kids do it.
- Get off the elevator two floors before your stop and

climb the stairs the rest of the way. (*Note:* Don't do this unless you are in good health.)
- Hang the laundry out on a line instead of putting it in the dryer.
- When you're going to take the bus, walk past your regular stop and get on board two or three blocks down the line.

The possibilities for burning more calories are practically endless, and you'll think of many more ways to incorporate the technique into your life. Of course, sometimes you will be limited by time constraints. Doing things the hard way often means doing things the long way. Nevertheless, the results over days and weeks will be worth it.

DAY 6 LUNCH
Today's lunch, like yesterday's, can be almost sumptuous. Start with a serving of hot cabbage soup, then have as much grilled, broiled, or roasted chicken or grilled or broiled fish as you like, as well as a salad of leafy greens and other vegetables.

AFTERNOON BLAHS OR BLUES?
With all the high-protein foods you've been eating today, you may not need to recharge with a midday snack. If you do begin to feel draggy, have more chicken or fish, or some higher-sugar vegetables, such as carrots. Don't forget the instant lift you get from the caffeine in tea or coffee.

STRESS RELIEF
Late in the diet, some people begin to feel stressed out. It can feel like hunger, it can feel like a food craving (they're different, as you know from reading through the chapter for Day 5). But often the feelings of stress are linked to what some diet experts call the need for "food soothing." This

need strikes particularly hard at those dieters who have learned to use food and eating to relieve stress, calm nerves, and reduce tension. Often the longer the need for food soothing is denied, the stronger it becomes.

Calming with Deep Breathing

Deep breathing can bring you tremendous nonfood stress relief. Here's how to do it:

1. With your chest lifted high, sit or stand up straight and take several deep breaths. Inhale slowly through your nose. As you inhale, concentrate on expanding your diaphragm—the muscular wall separating your chest from your stomach. Try to fill up that area with air. Don't gasp, puff out your chest, or suck in your gut when you inhale.
2. Hold your breath for an instant. Then exhale slowly through your mouth.

The idea is to breathe in and out a bit more slowly and deeply than you ordinarily do. If you do it properly, you can benefit from calming deep breathing anytime, anywhere, without calling attention to yourself.

You might recognize the technique as the same one many performing artists use to calm preperformance nerves. It will work for you, too. The effects are only temporary, of course. But you will discover that taking several deep breaths when the need for food soothing strikes will ease tension long enough to give you a chance to collect yourself and get your priorities back in order.

DAY 6 DINNER

Begin, as always, with a large serving of hot cabbage soup. Have a main course of more chicken or fish. If you're tired of grilled or broiled fish, try poaching it. (The general principles are on page 75 of chapter 5.) Add free veggies, as much and as many as you like. Today, like yesterday, is dessertless, but by the time you finish everything on your plate, you'll be too full for it anyway!

Reminder: Finish your yogurt or skim milk now unless you want to have it before you go to bed.

NONFOOD TREAT TIME

Many dieters are most vulnerable to the need for food soothing on the last day or so of the diet, so this is the perfect time to get out of the house and into an entertaining nonfood environment. If there's a ballet company, orchestra, music group, stage play, or sporting event you're eager to see, call about ticket availability. (Except for truly major events, you'll probably be able to get seats.) A long, lavish bubble bath is a natural soother as well.

Otherwise, repeat one of the activities that gave you pleasure earlier in the diet, or turn to chapter 6 for more ideas.

READY FOR SHUT-EYE

Get out your diet journal and applaud yourself and the progress you made today. Don't write about the fact that tomorrow is the last day of the diet. It's still too soon to anticipate the end. Treat today, instead, as just one more step in the process—one more day in which you behaved with confidence and conviction. One more *successful* day.

CHAPTER 17

Day 7

You probably woke up in a mood that is nothing short of triumphant. This is, after all, your final day on the New Cabbage Soup Diet, and you may have the heady feeling of a winner on a roll. No wonder: You *are* a winner. You've earned that natural high!

Perhaps you're surprised that just following a diet to its conclusion could make you feel this good. But think about it again, and you'll realize that what you are feeling is more than just the elation of having been successful so far into the plan. You're also feeling the excitement of being in charge and taking responsibility. You *know* that if you can do what you set out to do where dieting is concerned, you can do almost anything.

In some ways, this final day of the diet will seem familiar. That's because the food you'll be eating on Day 7 is essentially the same as what you had on Day 3. No more surprises. You've been through the complete food cycle and now you're almost back to where you started—minus up to ten pounds, and maybe even more!

Reminder: Don't start the day without reading this chapter from beginning to end. It's packed with tips and information that will ease you through the last day.

THE NEW CABBAGE SOUP DIET, DAY 7

On the menu today:
Unlimited cabbage soup
Unlimited free fruits
Unlimited free vegetables
1 8-ounce serving skim milk or plain, no-fat yogurt
Tea or coffee, plain or with artificial sweetener
Water
1 tablespoon low-fat, low-cal salad dressing
Your choice of herbs, spices, and other low-cal or
      no-cal flavoring ingredients

WAKE UP AND WRITE

You probably can hardly wait to step on the scale. But don't
do it. The final results of the New Cabbage Soup Diet aren't
in yet. Tomorrow morning you'll *really* have something to
crow about. For now, reach for your diet journal and give
yourself all the credit you deserve. Use positive self-talk
and don't dwell on the thought that it's your last day on
the diet. Write about your commitment to weight loss as if
today is just one more step in the journey toward achieving
the slimmer, healthier body you want for yourself.

BREAKFAST!

Naturally sweet and luscious flavors were missing from
Days 5 and 6, and you're probably eager for fruit again.
Treat yourself to the freshest, ripest ones in the refrigerator.
You're allowed as much fruit as you want, which means
that you can enjoy two, three, or more varieties. Have them
separately or in a fruit salad, with or without plain, no-fat
yogurt. *Reminder:* If you start out with yogurt for breakfast, you are not permitted to switch to skim milk later in
the day. If you haven't yet tried broiled fruit, why not do
so today? To enhance the natural goodness, sprinkle on a

few grains of artificial sweetener after you remove the fruit from the broiler.

MINI-WORKOUT

Walk, jog in place, give the easy "weight-lifting" exercises from Day 5 another try. Or just get up and dance. That's right, dance. Turn on the radio and surf the dial until you find music that makes you want to shimmy, swing, sway, twist, shuffle, hop, bounce, glide, whatever. Really get into it. Move your entire body, not just your feet and legs. Don't worry about what the kids, your spouse, or your house-mates might think. Everyone dances in private once in a while. Dance as long as time allows or until you feel slightly winded.

Reminder: Yesterday you learned about the weight-loss advantages of doing things the hard way. It's more than just a good idea for dieters; it's a weight-control technique that can help thin people maintain their weight and help every-one else control it.

KEEP IT UP

Do more exercise, rather than less, when you finish this cycle of the New Cabbage Soup Diet. Whether you plan to come back to this diet again (remember, you must wait at least fourteen days before you start the diet again) or decide to go on to a slower, long-term diet—or just want to main-tain the weight loss you've achieved over the last seven days—exercise will help. Plan to make it part of your life from now on.

The super-easy mini-workouts in this section were de-signed to introduce you to the concept of being more active, to help ease you into the habit of including more activity in your daily schedule, as well as to burn off just a few more calories than you might otherwise do. You will need to do a lot more exercise—especially of the aerobic kind—

to attain true fitness and the health and weight-control benefits it confers, and chapter 20 will help get you started.

DAY 7 LUNCH
A serving of hot cabbage soup and plenty of free fruit and vegetables is what you'll have today. Include yogurt (if today is a yogurt day for you), or finish with a glass of skim milk.

Reminder: Today's lunch can be as nutritious, healthful, and as filling as you want it to be since you can eat as much soup, vegetables, and fruit as you want. Still, after two days of protein-laden lunches, today's midday meal might leave you with the feeling that something is missing. To make sure you get the maximum in terms of satisfaction and enjoyment, turn back to chapter 9 and review the tips that help you get "more bang for the bite."

P.M. PICKUPS
If you need revitalizing this afternoon, have more fruit. As you know, the natural sugars in fruit can help raise blood sugar levels and quickly pep you up again. Try tea or coffee for an extra-energy boost.

Reminder: If at all possible, stop what you are doing for a few minutes in the middle of the afternoon and go outdoors for a quick walk. Brisk movement is one of the best antidotes for midafternoon energy drain. Stretching the large muscles of your body is almost as good, so if you can't get out of the building, try the simple stretching techniques described in chapter 12.

THE BOREDOM FACTOR
The New Cabbage Soup Diet is designed for quick weight loss, which is why it's made up almost entirely of low-calorie, low-fat, high-fiber soup, fruits, and vegetables, with a few other foods—such as skim milk and yogurt and the

animal protein on Days 5 and 6—to round it out. But by the time you reach Day 7, boredom with this strict and structured regimen can set in.

Boredom—with the food, with the routine, even with the constant need to maintain self-discipline—is one of the biggest challenges on this and other quick weight-loss plans in which food is necessarily limited in variety as well as calories. (Boredom can be a problem even on a longer-term diet that includes foods from all the food groups, but not as much of them as you have been accustomed to.) The following simple tips for coping with diet boredom will help get you through today and any day that diet boredom begins to get you down.

- *Shake up your schedule.* Anything you can do to relieve the sameness and regimentation of other parts of your life will help with diet boredom, too. If you are at work, arrange to finish what you're doing and leave early, if possible, so you can take in a mid-afternoon movie, drive out to the beach, visit a museum or art gallery, or spend some unplanned intimate hours with your spouse or lover. If you've been shut up in the house, get out. If you've been keeping to yourself, seek company.

- *Get busy.* Although it's not as much fun as sneaking off to a movie or making love, tackling the things that need to be done is another way to banish boredom. Answer mail, make those phone calls you've been putting off, update your to-do list. If you're at home, reorganize a closet, put all those photographs in an album at last, clean out the garage. Any work that keeps your brain or your body fully occupied will also make time fly and take your mind off food and diet.

- *Try positive imaging.* This is similar to positive self-talk, but instead of using words and phrases, you're going to work with mental pictures. If you do it correctly, escaping into a brief, very pleasurable fantasy can do away with boredom almost as well as the real thing. Here's how:

1. Sit or lie down in the most comfortable position you can manage. With your eyes closed, take ten deep, slow breaths. Try to make your mind a blank.

2. When you are thoroughly relaxed, conjure up the most gratifying images of yourself you can think of. For many dieters, the best thing imaginable is a mental scenario in which they are pounds slimmer and looking and feeling their best. Others prefer to imagine the realization of some other goal, such as a special career success, getting engaged, having a baby. Still others fantasize about being in the movies . . . even winning the lottery! The content of your fantasy is less important than its power to carry you away, so make the fantasy as vivid and detailed as you can.

3. After five minutes, bring yourself back to the real world—but try to keep the excitement and pleasurable feeling of the fantasy wrapped around you as you continue with whatever you were doing before your session of positive imaging.

DAY 7 DINNER

With a little creativity today's dinner, with its unlimited amounts of soup, free vegetables, and fruit, can be a banquet. Start with a serving of hot cabbage soup, go on to a vegetable main dish and salad, finish with as much fresh, ripe fruit as you want. You'll find many ideas for flavoring each in chapter 9.

Reminder: Finish your yogurt or skim milk now unless you'd rather have it as a bedtime snack.

NONFOOD TREAT TIME

Just because it's your last day on the diet doesn't mean you can skip this important part of the weight-loss routine. As you probably are beginning to realize, doing something pleasurable as a reward for abiding by the rules of the diet does more than keep you motivated and committed. It also helps you recognize that you can have fun and enjoy yourself without resorting to food. That's one of the most important lessons you can learn on the New Cabbage Soup Diet.

DAY'S END, DIET'S OVER

You did it! It's the last part of the final day of this seven-day diet, and you came through like a champ. Congratulations. You probably feel like celebrating—and for good reason—but it's too late in the day for that, so reach for your diet journal and give yourself all the praise you deserve—a figurative ticker tape parade down Broadway! Believe it or not, the excitement you feel tonight is nothing to what you'll experience tomorrow when you step on the bathroom scale.

THE END . . . AND A NEW BEGINNING

Now is a good time to reflect on the diet, on your feelings about your seven-day success story, and on your future. Put it all down on paper, along with your intentions regarding further weight loss.

You have many options. Although you must end this cycle of the New Cabbage Soup Diet now because it's too low-cal and limited for long-term use, you can go back to it after two weeks or more of healthy, well-balanced eating. Or you might prefer to start on a sensible, slower-working diet that includes a greater variety of food, and use the New Cabbage Soup Diet as a once-in-a-while tool for accelerating weight loss. Or instead of "dieting," you can work hard at changing your everyday eating habits for good. More and more experts in the field of weight loss recommend the latter, and you'll find important information on how to make lasting changes in chapter 20.

The one thing you definitely should not do, if you care about your health and your weight, is go back to your old way of eating—the one that created the problem that made you try this diet in the first place. Have some of your favorite foods tomorrow if you want them, but promise yourself: no binges. No filling up on high-fat meals and snacks. Nothing that will undo the good results you've achieved on this diet. It shouldn't be hard. After all, you've already proved to yourself how disciplined and in control you are . . . and you already know you're a success.

CHAPTER 18

Day 8 and After: How to Stay on Track

Here you are, flushed with success the day after completing your first seven-day New Cabbage Soup Diet cycle. It's time to see what you've accomplished. Slip out of your clothes, step on the scale, and record your new weight in your diet journal. Check your measurements and record them, too.

The total number of pounds and inches you lost will have had a lot to do with how faithful you were to the rules of the diet, as well as with how much you weighed when you started the diet.

In general, the more overweight you are, the greater the number of pounds you will lose in your first seven-day cycle. The original version of the diet projected a loss of seventeen pounds in a week! The men and women who actually do lose that astonishing amount are, typically, sixty pounds or more overweight (as measured by standard height/weight charts) when they start the diet. A loss of up to ten pounds—the amount mentioned throughout this book—is typical for men and women who are less than sixty pounds over normal weight when they begin the diet.

But whatever their starting weight, most people who abide by all the rules of the diet are not just surprised when the final results are in, they're elated. Some are so thrilled, so motivated—and experience such exuberant feelings of confidence—that they want to go right back to Day 1 of the diet and start all over again. Maybe you feel the same way.

Don't do it. It has been said many times elsewhere in this book and it's worth repeating here: You must wait at least two weeks after completing one New Cabbage Soup Diet cycle before beginning another.

TIME TO RECOUP

Your body needs a change from this very low-cal, low-fat, high-fiber regimen. The New Cabbage Soup Diet supplies your body with many good, healthful foods. But as you know from having read previous chapters, this diet does not give you adequate amounts of *all* the nutrients you need for optimal nutrition.

Two weeks of sensible eating that includes more of the foods that are in short supply on the diet—such as calcium-rich, low-fat dairy products, whole grains, and small amounts of healthful fats and oils such as olive oil, canola oil, and other vegetable oils—will give your body a chance to catch up on its nutritional needs.

It's worth repeating. Don't return to the diet until two weeks have elapsed. Instead, use the two weeks to help yourself to a slimmer, healthier future by changing your eating habits.

In chapter 19, you will find what hundreds of Cabbage Soup dieters have been waiting for: the New Cabbage Soup Maintenance Plan, complete with recipes, menus, and tips for adapting it to the way you live your life.

But don't skip the pages that follow. They're packed with information and food guidelines that you can use whether you intend to move on to the New Cabbage Soup Maintenance Plan or prefer to customize your own plan for healthy eating.

NOT TO LECTURE, BUT . . .

It's axiomatic. If you don't want to gain back the pounds you have just lost, you can't go back to your old way of eating. The point is so obvious, it hardly seems worth mentioning. Yet so many dieters—and not just the ones who have successfully completed the New Cabbage Soup Diet— fail to "get it." They lose pounds and inches, then revert to the eating patterns that made them overweight in the first place. When the pounds start to pile on again, they say the diet didn't work.

Most diets *do* work. Meaning that if you are not handicapped by genetic factors that make you super-resistant to weight loss, you can lose pounds on almost any food plan that supplies your body with fewer calories than it burns off during the day.

The New Cabbage Soup Diet gives you amazing, quick results. Other diets work more slowly. But no matter what diet you use to lose weight, you will gain it back again if you do not change your eating habits for the better.

NUTRITION FIRST

In "reforming" your diet, goal one is to supply your body with all the nutrients it must have for good health. Basic principles of good nutrition have been condensed and published by the United States Department of Agriculture (USDA) in its Dietary Guidelines for Americans and Food Guide Pyramid.

You've probably seen the Food Guide Pyramid in magazines or newspapers or on TV, but for convenience's sake, the recommendations included with the Pyramid are given here:

Each Day
- Have 6 to 11 servings from the bread, pasta, rice, and cereal food group.
- Have 3 to 5 servings of vegetables.
- Have 2 to 4 servings of meat, poultry, fish, eggs, seeds, nuts, or dried beans or peas.
- Have 2 to 3 servings of fruit.

- Have 2 to 3 servings of milk, yogurt, cheese, or other dairy-based food.
- Eat fats, oils, and sweets only sparingly.

HOW TO CUSTOMIZE FOOD PYRAMID GUIDELINES

As you can see, there's plenty of leeway in the USDA dietary guidelines. The USDA suggests that you modify the guidelines according to your age, sex, and level of activity.

- **If you are a sedentary adult,** for example, you probably need only 6 servings from the bread, pasta, rice, and cereal group and 2 servings (for a total of 5 ounces) from the meat, poultry, fish, and other proteins group.
- **If you are an active woman or moderately active man,** 9 servings from the bread, pasta, rice, and cereal group and 2 servings (for a total of 6 ounces) from the meat, poultry, fish, and other proteins group would be sufficient.
- **If you are a very active man,** you may require the full 11 servings of bread, pasta, rice, and cereal and the full 3 servings (for a total of 7 ounces) from the meat, poultry, and other proteins group.

CONTROL THOSE PORTIONS

Even correcting for sex and activity levels, the Dietary Guidelines for Americans would seem to encourage eating huge amounts of food. However, a "serving" is probably smaller than you think.

The USDA definitions of a serving of various types of food are listed below. Adhering to these definitions will help you get great results on the New Cabbage Soup Diet Maintenance Plan as well as on any other weight-loss or weight-maintenance program you might decide to try.

Bread, Pasta, Rice, Cereals

A serving of bread is 1 slice; a serving of cooked cereal, rice, or pasta, is ½ cup; a serving of ready-to-eat cereal is 1 cup.

Vegetables

A serving of raw, leafy vegetables is 1 cup (loosely packed); a serving of other vegetables is ½ cup; a serving of vegetable juice is ¾ cup.

Fruit

A serving of fruit is 1 medium apple, banana, orange, or other fresh fruit of comparable size; a serving of chopped, cooked, or canned fruit is ½ cup; a serving of fruit juice is ¾ cup.

Meat, Poultry, Fish, Eggs, Nuts, Dried Beans

A serving of lean meat, poultry, or fish is 2 to 3 ounces: a serving of cooked dried beans or peas is ½ cup. One egg or 2 tablespoons peanut butter or ⅓ cup nuts or ½ cup tofu count as 1 ounce of lean meat.

Milk, Yogurt, Cheese

A serving of milk or yogurt is 1 cup; a serving of "natural" (not processed) cheese is 1½ ounces; a serving of processed cheese is 2 ounces.

Fats, Oils, and Sweets

There are no serving sizes given for fats, oils, and sweets. Instead, the USDA advises you to go easy on the butter, margarine, gravy, salad dressing, sugar, and jelly you add to food in cooking or at the table and to choose lower-fat and lower-sugar prepared foods. You also are advised to avoid greasy or highly sweetened snack foods and to avoid or limit sweetened soft drinks.

CUT THE FAT

Simply eating according to USDA guidelines might be enough to keep your weight stable. If the needle on the bathroom scale does start to inch up more than a pound or so, another round of New Cabbage Soup Diet eating—either the seven-day or three-day blitz version—should bring your weight back to where you want it.

But whether the goal is weight stabilization or weight loss, for your health's sake, you should make an effort to reduce food fat.

- Cook with less fat or no fat. This means broiling, grilling, steaming, poaching, or simmering rather than deep-frying. It also means using less fat in sautéing and browning. Skillets with nonstick coatings are a big help here. They make it possible to sauté many foods with just a vegetable oil cooking spray. You may need to use some oil to sauté certain foods or to brown meats, but with a nonstick skillet, you can use less than you would if you were using ordinary cookware.
- When preparing foods such as pasta, stuffings, and sauces from scratch or from a packaged mix, use less fat than the directions call for. In most cases, the dish you are making will be just as successful and taste just as good if you use only half the oil or fat specified in the instructions.
- Use lower-fat or skim milk in recipes calling for cream. Except where cream is necessary to create a thick, rich consistency, you'll get the same good results but with fewer calories. (Did you know? Chilled, evaporated skim milk can be whipped, like cream!)
- Substitute plain, low-fat, or no-fat yogurt for sour cream as a topping or in recipes.
- When you shop for meat, choose the leanest cuts. Trim all visible fat from meat and poultry before you

cook it. Discard the skin before you serve chicken or turkey.

- Use little or no butter or margarine, commercial salad dressing, or mayonnaise on vegetables and other food. Flavor with lemon juice and fresh herbs instead. The exception: Try drizzling a small amount of healthful olive oil on vegetables. Delicious! And your body will appreciate the essential fatty acids.

- Choose lower-fat versions of yogurt, milk, cheese, frozen desserts, processed meat, such as bologna, salami, and ham, and other products. However, keep in mind that even these lower-fat foods are high in calories and will add unwanted pounds if you eat too much of them.

KNOW "FRIENDLY" FATS FROM FATTY FOES

If you've been eating the standard American diet, you'll benefit by cutting your fat intake. In cutting the fat, you will be taking in fewer calories, and, if you've been getting much of your fat from animal sources, you'll be lowering your risk for a range of diseases.

But we all need *some* fat—specifically, the essential fatty acids necessary for good health and for life itself. Certain fats are better than others and actually have been shown to lower heart disease risk. So know your fats, and choose wisely.

Saturated Fats—Avoid Them

Saturated fats are those that are solid at room temperature. Most come from animal sources. These fats raise cholesterol levels, and as you know, high blood cholesterol is a risk factor for heart disease. To reduce saturated fats in your diet, eat less of the following.

- Fatty meats
- Lard

- Cheese and other dairy products, including whole milk, yogurt, and sour cream
- Foods made with coconut and palm oils, which are also high in saturated fats

When you have a choice, substitute unsaturated fats for saturated.

Unsaturated fats—Always Better Choices!

Fats that are liquid at room temperature tend to be high in unsaturated fats—both monounsaturated and polyunsaturated—and are derived primarily from plant sources. Both monounsaturated and polyunsaturated fats tend to lower blood cholesterol levels, decreasing your risk for heart disease.

Common sources of *monounsaturated* fats are:

- Olive oil
- Peanut oil
- Canola oil

The following oils are high in *polyunsaturated* fats:

- Corn oil
- Soybean oil
- Sunflower oil

Here are easy ways to get more of the good fats (and less of the bad fats) into your diet:

- Read labels. Whenever possible, choose products made with the polyunsaturated fats, mentioned above. Avoid products containing saturated fats. (Remember, although coconut and palm oils are vegetable in origin, they are high in saturated fats.)
- When you have a choice, cook with vegetable oil instead of butter, lard, or other animal fats.

- Choose salad dressings made with pure vegetable oils such as olive oil.

Remember, *some* fat is essential for good health, but even the "good" fats are high in calories and should be used sparingly.

CREATE A CUSTOMIZED DIET FOR SLOW, STEADY WEIGHT LOSS

The Food Guide Pyramid is a solid foundation on which to base an individualized weight-loss plan. The trick is to customize it so that it "fits" your body and your food preferences.

Calculate Your Calorie Needs

To estimate the number of calories you can eat each day without gaining or losing weight, start by multiplying your current weight by one of the following numbers:

> If you are a sedentary man: multiply by 16.
> If you are a sedentary woman: multiply by 14.
>
> If you are a somewhat active man: multiply by 18.
> If you are a somewhat active woman: multiply by 16.
>
> If you are an active man: multiply by 21.
> If you are an active woman: multiply by 18.

Let's say you're a man who spends most of every day at a desk and makes little or no effort to exercise. Your current weight is 160 pounds. To find the number of calories you need each day to maintain your current weight, multiply 160 by 16 (because you are sedentary).

$$160 \times 16 = 2,560$$

Now you know that to avoid weight gain or weight loss, you need to consume approximately 2,560 calories each day.

But what if you want to lose weight? If that's the case, you need to consume fewer than 2,560 calories daily. All else being equal, if you reduced your calorie intake by 100 each day, you would lose about 10 pounds in a year. Reducing your calories by 200 would result in a 20-pound loss over a year. And so on.

Of course, you might want to recalculate as you lose weight. Let's say you started at 160 pounds and have lost 10 pounds over the last few months but have not increased your activity level. To find out how many calories you can consume and continue to lose weight at the same slow rate, multiply your new weight, 150 pounds, by 16.

$$150 \times 16 = 2,400$$

Now that you've lost 10 pounds, 2,400 calories per day is the new magic number to aim for if you want to continue to lose weight at about the same rate.

Note: These figures are approximate. The actual number of calories you require to maintain your weight or lose pounds will vary depending on your age, your metabolic inheritance, increases and decreases in activity levels, and other factors. Nevertheless, the formula provides a good starting point for planning a diet that produces slow, steady weight loss, and you can always adjust your calorie intake up or down if need be.

PUTTING IT ALL TOGETHER

Now you have much of the information you need to create a plan for maintaining your current weight or for losing pounds gradually over weeks and months.

- Use Food Guide Pyramid suggestions as your foundation for good nutrition.

- Use the fat-cutting tips to pare away unnecessary calories.
- Use the formula for calculating the number of calories you need to keep your weight stable or to lose pounds slowly and steadily.

Finally, adjust your food intake so that you are consuming the number of calories necessary for maintenance or weight loss. How do you manage that? Read food labels to find the calories per serving of prepared foods. Get a book that lists the calorie content of a wide variety of other foods and consult it regularly. (You'll soon know the approximate numbers of calories in common foods by heart.) Eat less of the higher-calorie foods and more of the ones containing fewer calories.

Complicated? Not really. Like many things in life, healthful eating is easier in practice than reading about it. Use these principles in good health. Want still more guidance? See how it all plays out in the Cabbage Soup Maintenance Plan.

CHAPTER 19

The New Cabbage Soup Maintenance Plan

Okay, you lost pounds in a hurry on the New Cabbage Soup Diet. More congratulations are in order! In the previous chapter, you learned basic principles for maintaining your new weight and for creating a food plan you can live with for the rest of your life. The information in that chapter was included in the first New Cabbage Soup Diet book, and many readers responded positively to the idea of devising a customized diet for weight maintenance and weight loss.

But some readers wanted more. They wanted information that went beyond generalities to include specifics. They wanted meal plans, they wanted recipes. And they wanted it all keyed to the New Cabbage Soup Diet—the amazing weight-loss plan that had given them such extraordinary results.

So here it is, by popular demand, the New Cabbage Soup Maintenance Plan. Let's start with soup, a major component of the plan, and go on from there to meal-by-meal suggestions and guidelines.

SOUP . . . STILL THE KEY

Cabbage soup, as you know from your own experience on the diet, is uniquely satisfying and filling. Research confirms the effectiveness of soup as an aid to weight control, as we saw back in chapter 2, which cites a study showing that soup before a meal decreases appetite and makes weight loss (and weight maintenance, which is the goal here) easier. In fact, soup is an ideal weight-control tool. That is why healthy, nutrient-packed, low-cal soup, the foundation of the diet, also plays an important role in the Cabbage Soup Maintenance Plan.

On this plan, as on the diet, you are encouraged to have as much cabbage soup as you like, any time of day or night. Have it at lunch, at dinner, between meals, at bedtime. Use it as a substitute for high-cal, high-fat, low-nutrition junk food when the craving for something to eat begins to get to you. Put it to work for you. Let it do what it was meant to do: Fill you up with low-cal nutrients, stave off hunger and food cravings, and help you maintain your weight— just as it helped you lose weight on the diet.

But one of the important differences between the New Cabbage Soup Diet and the maintenance plan is that on the diet, you were directed to make cabbage soup a part of every meal. On the maintenance plan, cabbage soup is no longer a several-times-a-day "must." Instead, it's an option, ready whenever you need it to help you control your eating.

CABBAGE SOUP ALTERNATIVES

Cabbage soup is great tasting, rich in nutrients, and super-satisfying. Whoever created the original Cabbage Soup Diet recognized its usefulness as an aid to weight loss and made it the star of the diet. But, in fact, cabbage soup is not the world's only nutritious, low-cal soup. And although its status as ace fat fighter remains unchallenged, on the maintenance plan, you are invited to alternate the basic cabbage soup with your choice of any number of tasty, healthful soups. In fact, you can use almost any low-cal, low-fat soup to kick off your meals and help you control your weight. There are dozens of different soups that fill the bill.

Super Soups to Try

For starters, you can use prepared canned or packaged soups from the supermarket. Read and compare labels to find the ones that are lowest in calories and fat.

Soups from the Supermarket

Choose: clear chicken or beef broth or consommé, onion soup, tomato soup (if condensed, dilute with water or low-fat milk), vegetable soups, chicken-vegetable or beef-vegetable soups, Manhattan (tomato-based) clam chowder. (Many of these soups are available in reduced fat and/or low-sodium versions.)

Avoid: creamed soups, cheese soups, bean soups, mostly noodle Asian soups.

SOUPS YOU MAKE

Impromptu Soups

You don't have to be a kitchen whiz to throw together a tasty, nutritious pot of soup. All it takes is an adventurous spirit, some soup stock—chicken, beef, or vegetable-flavor bouillon cubes or packets will do, as will canned chicken or beef broth, bottled clam juice, or even plain water—and a few odds and ends. Exact amounts are unimportant. Here are a few guidelines:

- Dissolve bouillon cubes or granules in water according to package instructions. (Or start with canned broth or canned broth mixed with tomato or vegetable juice. Use clam juice if you want to make clam or fish chowder. If you have none of the above on hand, or if other soup ingredients are particularly flavorful, use plain water.)
- Add a few vegetables. These can be leftovers from a

previous meal, canned or frozen veggies, or you can raid the fridge for fresh vegetables. (Chopped onions, minced garlic, chopped celery, sliced carrots, and sliced mushrooms are always good choices, but don't stop there. Green beans, canned or fresh tomatoes, squash, peas, chopped spinach, escarole or other leafy greens . . . any or all of these can go into an impromptu soup.)

- Toss in bits of leftover meat or chicken if you have them. (For chowder, add chopped fresh or canned clams or other seafood.)
- At this point, you might need to adjust the ratio of stock (liquid) to other ingredients and add more stock if necessary.
- Sprinkle in some dried or chopped fresh herbs, such as thyme, basil, or oregano.
- Simmer until the soup is hot. (If you are using fresh vegetables, simmer until they are tender.)
- Optional: Stir in ½ cup or so of leftover rice or pasta during the last few minutes of cooking time.
- Season with salt, pepper, herbs, or spices. If you want stronger flavor, try adding a few drops of Worcestershire sauce or hot sauce. Enjoy!

Not *that* adventurous? Then here are three easy soup recipes for you to try.

Very Vegetable Soup

- 2 large onions, coarsely chopped
- 6 stalks celery, sliced
- 6 to 7 carrots, sliced
- 2 cups spinach, coarsely chopped
- 1½ cups green beans, sliced into bite-size pieces
- 2 large cloves garlic, minced
- 1 bay leaf

- 3 quarts water
- Salt and pepper

Combine ingredients in a large pot and bring to a boil. Reduce heat to a simmer, cover the pot, and cook for about an hour or until carrots and beans are tender. Season with salt and pepper to taste.

Tomato-Mushroom-Onion Soup

- 2 large onions, coarsely chopped
- 2½ cups sliced fresh mushrooms
- 3 zucchini, cubed
- 2 large cloves garlic, minced
- 1½ tablespoons olive oil
- 3 16-ounce cans tomatoes
- 2 quarts water
- 2 bay leaves
- ½ teaspoon dried thyme
- Salt and pepper

In a large pot, sauté onions, mushrooms, zucchini, and garlic in olive oil until tender. Add tomatoes, water, bay leaves, and thyme. Cover the pot and simmer 20 minutes. Season with salt and pepper to taste.

Easy Onion Soup

- 5 cups onions, coarsely chopped
- 2 tablespoons olive oil
- 6 cups hot beef broth
- Salt and pepper to taste
- Parmesan cheese (optional)

Sauté the onions in olive oil until they are translucent. Stir into the beef broth. Season with salt and pepper. Top with Parmesan cheese before serving if desired.

Note: There are many good soup cookbooks out there. Since soup plays such an important role in the Cabbage Soup Maintenance Plan, you may want to invest in one. Look for a book that includes a selection of low-cal soups.

THE NEW CABBAGE SOUP MAINTENANCE PLAN—MEAL BY MEAL

In the following pages, you will find seven high-nutrition breakfasts, lunches, and dinners, plus ideas for snacks. These meals are heavy on fruits, vegetables, and grains. They supply lots of protein, only some of which comes from animal sources, and provide small amounts of fat, most of it "good," monounsaturated or polyunsaturated fat, which supplies essential fatty acids. (In some meals the fat is "hidden"—that is, it is an ingredient or nutritional component of one of the main foods on the menu.)

Many of the carbohydrate foods suggested here will help keep your blood sugar levels stable and prolong feelings of satiety after a meal.

You can use the menus that follow in the order given, or mix and match them at your convenience, or use them as models for creating meals that satisfy your own taste preferences.

The amounts of food specified in the Cabbage Soup Maintenance Plan menus are suggestions only and can be adjusted up or down to suit your age, sex, and activity level.

START WITH SOUP!

The rule for lunches and dinners is to start with soup—the key to maintaining your weight on this plan. Its role is to take the edge off your appetite while supplying you with vital nutrients, so don't skip it. Put it to work for you.

WAKE UP TO A HEALTHFUL BREAKFAST

Studies show that eating a healthful breakfast "jump starts" the brain and body after a long, eight-hour fast and adds

measurably to alertness and efficiency throughout the day.
Not only that, breakfast revs up metabolism first thing in
the morning and actually increases the rate of calorie burn-
off for hours afterward. Throw in the fact that without
breakfast, you are going to be more vulnerable to the lure
of high-fat, high-cal items later on, and you can see why
eating breakfast is always a good idea.

On the New Cabbage Soup Maintenance Plan, you will
be eating breakfast every day—a real breakfast (not just
coffee and orange juice) that gets you off to the best possible start, makes sense in nutritional terms, and delays
hunger.

The seven days' worth of breakfast menus are listed in
no particular order. You can try them all, or, if you are a
creature of habit, you can have the same breakfast over and
over again until you are ready for a change. (The exception
is Breakfast #4, which includes an egg. Because eggs are
relatively high in cholesterol, many doctors advise limiting
eggs to no more than three per week.)

Breakfast #1

    Whole-grain cereal (Look for one that is vitamin
           enriched and has 3 to 5 grams of fiber and no
           more than 8 grams of sugar per serving.)
    Banana
    8 ounces low-fat milk (use some on your cereal)
    Coffee or tea if desired

Breakfast #2

    Broiler "Cheese Danish"
    (Toast 1 slice of bread, preferably whole grain;
           spread with cottage cheese, sprinkle with
           cinnamon and a small amount of sugar, and
           place under the broiler until bubbly.)
    ½ grapefruit
    8 ounces low-fat milk
    Coffee or tea if desired

Breakfast #3

    1 cup plain yogurt topped with

    Wheat germ and

    Pineapple chunks (fresh pineapple is preferable;
        canned is fine, but rinse it first, if it was
        packed in syrup)

    8 ounces low-fat milk

    Coffee or tea if desired

Breakfast #4

    1 egg boiled or scrambled in a small amount of
        olive oil served on

    Whole-grain bread toasted

    ½ cantaloupe or other melon

    8 ounces low-fat milk

    Coffee or tea if desired

Breakfast #5

    3 ounces water-pack tuna or sardines spiked with
        lemon juice

    1 tomato sliced (run it under the broiler for extra
        goodness, if you have the time)

    Whole-grain bread toasted

    8 ounces low-fat milk

    Coffee or tea if desired

Breakfast #6

    Hot oatmeal

    Apple slices spread with peanut butter

    8 ounces low-fat milk

    Coffee or tea if desired

Breakfast #7

    French toast

    (1 slice whole-grain bread soaked in egg beaten
        with a drop or two of vanilla extract and
        lightly browned in a skillet; sprinkle with

> cinnamon and a small amount of sugar before
> serving)
¾ cup orange juice
8 ounces low-fat milk
Coffee or tea if desired

MIDMORNING SNACK ATTACK

A midmorning snack is not a must on the Cabbage Soup Maintenance Plan, but if you feel the need for a quick energy and pickup before lunch, go ahead, have something to eat. Choose one of the following:

- Cabbage soup, as much as you like
- Fruit, 1 piece of any of the free fruits listed in chapter 5
- Raw or cooked vegetables, 1 cup of any of the free vegetables listed in chapter 5
- Rice cake spread with peanut butter or unsweetened fruit spread
- Scant handful of almonds or peanuts
- Fat-free yogurt
- Vegetable juice

EAT A POWER LUNCH

The amount and kind of food you eat at lunch has an enormous influence on how you will feel and perform during the afternoon—as well as on how well you control your eating for the rest of the day. We have all had the experience of consuming too much high-cal, high-fat food at lunch and feeling stuffed, sluggish, and sleepy for hours afterward. In fact, some studies have shown that even moderate amounts of the wrong foods can have a negative effect on mental and physical performance in the afternoon, while eating certain other foods can boost performance.

For example, in one study, two groups of volunteers were given two different lunches. One group got pasta with tomato sauce and bread. The other group received a smaller amount of pasta and a portion of lean turkey. The two lunches supplied equal numbers of calories. After lunch, all volunteers were given tests to assess alertness and ability to concentrate. Results: The volunteers who ate the pasta-and-turkey lunch performed measurably better and continued to perform better for a full two hours after lunch.

On the Cabbage Soup Maintenance Plan, you will be eating lunches that keep you alert, energized, and on top of things, without adding excess calories to your day's total.

Lunch on the plan always starts with a soup, either cabbage soup or one of the low-fat, low-cal soups (bought or homemade) suggested earlier. Lunches also include carbohydrates, protein, and a small amount of fat.

Remember, you can use these sample menus below as is or as models for planning healthy lunches that take into account your individual food preferences.

Lunch #1

  Cabbage soup or other low-cal, low-fat soup
  Salad of lettuce, tomato, onion rings, and sliced
    turkey dressed with small amount of vinegar
    and olive oil
  Whole-grain bread
  Coffee or tea if desired

Lunch #2

  Cabbage soup or other low-cal, low-fat soup
  Hummus in pita pocket
  Bunch of grapes
  Coffee or tea if desired

Lunch #3

  Cabbage soup or other low-cal, low-fat soup
  Sushi
  Apple, pear, or other fresh fruit
  Coffee or tea if desired

Lunch #4
>Cabbage soup or other low-cal, low-fat soup
Baked potato topped with cottage cheese
Calcium-fortified orange juice
Coffee or tea if desired

Lunch #5
>Cabbage soup or other low-cal, low-fat soup
Pasta with clam sauce
Mango slices
Coffee or tea if desired

Lunch #6
>Cabbage soup or other low-cal, low-fat soup
Reduced-fat ham and cheese on whole-grain bread
Slice cantaloupe or other melon
Coffee or tea if desired

Lunch #7
>Cabbage soup or other low-cal, low-fat soup
Spinach, mushroom, and sliced hard-boiled egg
salad dressed with small amount of vinegar
and olive oil
Strawberries
Coffee or tea if desired

AFTERNOON PICKUP
Lunches on the plan may very well be enough to keep you going strong throughout the afternoon. However, if you do experience a three P.M. slowdown, try one of the midmorning snack suggestions mentioned earlier—and listed again here for your convenience:

- Cabbage soup, as much as you like
- Fruit, 1 piece of any of the free fruits listed in chapter 5

- Raw or cooked vegetables, 1 cup of any of the free vegetables listed in chapter 5
- Rice cake spread with peanut butter or unsweetened fruit spread
- Scant handful of almonds or peanuts
- Fat-free yogurt
- Vegetable juice

HAVE A HIGH-NUTRITION DINNER

Like lunches, dinners on the Cabbage Soup Maintenance Plan start with a steaming bowl of soup to take the edge off your appetite. Keep in mind that the amounts of food specified in these menus are suggestions only and can be adjusted up or down to suit your age, sex, and activity level.

Dinner #1

> Cabbage soup or other low-cal, low-fat soup
> Salad of lettuce, sliced oranges, and red onion rings dressed with a small amount of vinegar and olive oil
> Chicken Breast Roasted with Garlic*
> ½ cup brown rice
> ½ cup raspberry sorbet
> Coffee or tea if desired

*Chicken Breasts Roasted with Garlic

(4 servings)

- 4 chicken breasts, skin removed
- 2½ teaspoons dried sage
- Salt and pepper
- 3 tablespoons olive oil
- 2 whole heads garlic, separated into cloves (about 30), unpeeled
- 1 cup dry white wine

1. Preheat oven to 375°F. Sprinkle chicken with sage, salt, and pepper. Heat oil in a skillet over medium-high heat. Add chicken and sauté until brown, about 3 minutes per side.
2. Meanwhile, boil garlic in a small saucepan of water for 2 minutes. Then drain, rinse under cold water to cool, and peel.
3. Transfer chicken to a baking dish. Arrange garlic around chicken. Add wine. Cover the dish and bake for 10 to 12 minutes. Uncover and baste chicken with pan juices. Bake uncovered until cooked through, about 10 to 12 minutes longer, then transfer chicken to plates.
4. Boil pan juices over high heat until slightly thickened, about 2 minutes. Season with salt and pepper. Spoon garlic sauce over chicken and serve.

Dinner #2

Cabbage soup or other low-cal, low-fat soup
Green salad (use a mix of leafy greens such as lettuce, escarole, chicory, watercress; sprinkle with a scant handful of chopped black olives; dress with small amount of vinegar and olive oil)
Pasta with Tomato-Broccoli Sauce*
Broiled peaches
Coffee or tea if desired

*Pasta with Tomato-Broccoli Sauce

(4 servings)

Sauce

- 1 28-ounce can crushed tomatoes
- 2 cups steamed, fine-chopped broccoli florets
- 1½ teaspoons dried oregano
- 1½ teaspoons dried basil
- 2 cloves crushed garlic

- 8 ounces spaghetti or other pasta

- Salt and pepper to taste
- Parmesan or Romano cheese (optional)

1. Place tomatoes, steamed broccoli, oregano, basil, and garlic in a large saucepan. Simmer over low heat for about 30 minutes, stirring occasionally.
2. As sauce is heating, bring salted water to a boil in a large pot. Cook pasta according to package directions. Drain thoroughly when done.
3. Combine sauce and pasta, season with salt and pepper. Top with cheese if desired, and serve.

Dinner #3

Cabbage soup or other low-cal, low-fat soup
Shredded carrot, beet, and cabbage salad dressed
      with a small amount of vinegar and olive oil
Broiled Flounder Fillet*
Baked potato topped with plain yogurt and chopped
      chives
½ cup mixed fruit salad (your choice of sliced or
      chunked seasonal fruit)
Coffee or tea if desired

*Broiled Flounder Fillet

(4 servings)

- 1 onion chopped
- 2 cloves garlic, chopped
- 12 ounces filleted flounder
- Small amount vegetable oil
- Salt and pepper to taste
- 1 lemon, sliced in wedges

Sauté onion and garlic in vegetable oil until golden. Lightly grease a cookie sheet with vegetable oil. Place flounder on cookie sheet and broil until flesh is flaky. Sprinkle with onion and garlic. Season with salt and pepper. Serve with lemon wedges.

Dinner #4
> Cabbage soup or other low-cal, low-fat soup
> Pork, Onion, Green Pepper, and Mushroom Stir-Fry*
> Brown rice
> Frozen yogurt dessert
> Coffee or tea if desired

*Pork, Onion, Green Pepper, and Mushroom Stir-Fry

(4 servings)

- 2 tablespoons vegetable oil
- 12 ounces lean pork, cut into bite-size cubes
- 2 cups sliced green pepper
- 2 cups sliced onion
- 2 cups sliced mushrooms
- Salt, pepper, and soy sauce to taste

Heat the oil in a large skillet. Add pork and vegetables and sauté, stirring constantly, until pork is cooked through and vegetables are tender (about 15 minutes). Season with pepper and salt or soy sauce to taste.

Dinner #5
> Cabbage soup or other low-cal, low-fat soup
> Green Bean Salad*
> Grilled lean minute steak
> Whole-grain roll
> Slice angel food cake
> Coffee or tea if desired

*Green Bean Salad

(4 servings)

Dressing

- ½ cup plain nonfat yogurt
- ½ cup fat-free bottled Italian dressing
- 2 garlic cloves, chopped
- 1 tablespoon Dijon mustard
- 1 teaspoon Worcestershire sauce
- Fresh ground pepper to taste

- ½ pound green beans, rinsed and trimmed (use frozen if time is short)
- 1 head romaine lettuce, torn into bite-size pieces
- 2 tablespoons grated Parmesan cheese

1. Combine first five dressing ingredients in a small bowl. Stir briskly. Season with pepper.
2. Cook beans in boiling salted water until tender, about 5 minutes for fresh, less for frozen. Drain. Rinse with cold water and drain again. Combine beans, romaine lettuce, and cheese in a large bowl. Add dressing and toss.

Dinner #6

Cabbage soup or other low-cal, low-fat soup
Wilted escarole salad (steam escarole until slightly
softened; serve with small amount of vinegar
and olive oil
Easy Pita Pizza*
Ambrosia (orange and banana slices tossed with
unsweetened shredded coconut)
Coffee or tea if desired

*Easy Pita Pizza

(4 servings)

- 4 individual pita pockets, uncut
- ½ cup bottled pizza sauce
- ½ cup tomatoes, seeded and chopped
- ½ cup fresh mushrooms, chopped
- ½ teaspoon dried oregano
- 1 cup part-skin mozzarella cheese, shredded
- ¼ cup Parmesan cheese, grated

Preheat oven to 500°F. Arrange pitas on a baking sheet. Top with remaining ingredients. Bake for about 8 minutes or until crust is crisp.

Dinner #7

    Cabbage soup or other low-cal, low-fat soup
    Crudités (raw cauliflower, celery, carrots, and other
        vegetables, cut up and served with low-fat
        sour cream)
    Beefy Enchiladas*
    Sliced kiwifruit
    Coffee or tea if desired

*Beefy Enchiladas

(4 servings)

- ½ cup tomato sauce
- ½ cup bottled salsa
- 8 6-inch corn tortillas
- ½ pound lean ground beef
- 1 cup canned nonfat refried beans
- 1 teaspoon chili powder
- 1 teaspoon ground cumin
- ⅛ teaspoon black pepper
- ½ cup shredded reduced-fat cheddar cheese

1. In a small bowl, stir together tomato sauce and salsa. Using about half the tomato sauce mixture, brush both sides of each tortilla for flavor. Place tortillas on a plate and set aside.

2. In a large skillet, cook beef over medium-high heat until brown, about 5 minutes, stirring occasionally. Place beef in a colander and rinse under hot water to remove excess fat. Drain well. Wipe fat out of the skillet with a paper towel. Return beef to skillet. Stir in refried beans, chili powder, cumin, and pepper. Cook, stirring, for 2 minutes, or until heated through.

3. Preheat broiler. Spoon about ¼ cup of the mixture down the center of each tortilla. Roll up tortillas and place, seam side down, in a large glass baking dish. Top with remaining tomato sauce mixture. Broil 4 inches from the heat for 5 minutes, or until browned. Sprinkle with cheese. Let stand 5 minutes before serving.

There you have it, the Cabbage Soup Maintenance Plan— seven days of healthful, low-fat eating based on the unique diet that has helped thousands lose up to ten pounds in a week, look better, and feel better and more energized than ever before. The components are simple:

- High-nutrition breakfasts that jump-start your brain and prime your body for greater calorie burn-off throughout the day.
- Lunches and dinners that begin with nutritious, satisfying, low-cal soup—the key to safe, sure weight control—and include balanced amounts of carbohydrates, proteins, and a small amount of fat.
- Energy-boosting snacks that supply your body with even more of the essential nutrients it needs for optimal health.

Get a "feel" for the plan by using it as is, adjusting quantities and amounts according to your age, sex, activity levels, and calorie requirements, if necessary. Then use what you've learned to expand on the plan in the weeks and months to come.

CHAPTER 20

Get a Move On!

Throughout most of this book, the emphasis has been on how to use the New Cabbage Soup Diet for quick weight loss, whether you choose to exercise or not. But it's a fact that you will lose weight more surely and more rapidly—and you will look and feel even better, and perhaps even live longer—if you incorporate moderate exercise into your daily life. So let's shift the focus now to what you can do to be more active. The rewards—easier weight control and a healthier body—are definitely worth the effort.

KEEP IT UP!

As recently as twenty years ago, best-selling diet books rarely mentioned exercise as an ally in the fight against fat. When exercise was mentioned at all, it was often in the context of toning flabby muscles or defining a waistline, rather than as an aid to losing pounds or maintaining a healthy weight. Since then, studies measuring the impact of higher activity levels on dieters and nondieters alike have shown that exercise is indeed a useful tool for weight control.

For better heart health and overall fitness, the American Heart Association (AHA) suggests that everyone try to get in thirty to sixty minutes of vigorous physical activity three or four times a week. Later in this chapter, you will find suggestions and guidelines for starting and sticking to an exercise program that fulfills AHA goals. However, if you are struggling with a significant weight problem, you may not feel up to embarking on an ambitious exercise program just yet. That's okay. Instead, try to be just a little more active. *Some* exercise is always better than no exercise at all.

It was suggested in the diet days section of this book—chapters 11 through 17—that you try to get in just a few minutes of extra physical activity each day. The mini-workouts in those chapters contributed to calorie burn-off, helped to get you moving, and, it is hoped, accustomed you to the idea of setting aside time for exercise every day. Keep up those mini-workouts now, when you are between cycles of the New Cabbage Soup Diet or eating to maintain your weight on the maintenance plan. Even just a few minutes of extra activity each day can make a difference.

EVERYDAY WAYS TO BURN EXTRA CALORIES
Just doing things the hard way as you go about your life will burn extra calories and make weight control easier. Here are a few "hard" things you can do starting today.

- Do your own dusting, vacuuming, mopping, and other housework instead of hiring someone to do it for you. The same goes for gardening and lawn work.
- Whenever possible, walk briskly or ride a bike instead of driving.
- When you drive, park a few blocks away from your destination and walk briskly the rest of the way.
- Get off the elevator one or two floors before your stop, then use the stairs.

- Pace instead of standing still. (Got a cordless telephone? Walk while you talk.) Stand instead of sitting. Sit instead of lying down.
- Get up out of your chair to switch TV channels. (It has been estimated that in most homes, the walk from sofa to TV translates into an average of four miles a week!)
- At the office, use your feet instead of the intercom.
- Spend most of your lunch hour walking.

LITTLE THINGS COUNT

Remember, although frequent regular aerobic workouts should be your ultimate goal, any physical activity you engage in has value. The following chart shows the number of calories burned per hour for people of various weights during everyday activities.

ACTIVITY	120 lbs.	140 lbs.	160 lbs.	180 lbs.	200 lbs.	220 lbs.	240 lbs.	260 lbs.	280 lbs.	300 lbs.
Basketball, leisurely	156	182	208	234	260	286	312	338	364	390
Bowling	66	77	88	99	110	121	132	143	154	165
Dancing, freestyle	120	140	160	180	200	220	240	260	280	300
Dancing, slow	66	77	88	99	110	121	132	143	154	165
Gardening	108	126	144	162	180	198	216	234	252	270
Golfing, without a cart	120	140	160	180	200	220	240	260	280	300
Golfing, with a car	84	98	112	126	140	154	168	182	196	210
Ironing	60	70	80	90	100	110	120	130	140	150
Mopping	102	119	136	153	170	187	204	221	238	255
Mowing the lawn	162	189	216	243	270	297	324	351	378	405
Ping Pong	108	126	144	162	180	198	216	234	252	270
Raking leaves	90	105	120	135	150	165	180	195	210	225
Scrubbing the floor	168	196	224	252	280	308	336	364	392	420
Shopping	72	84	96	108	120	132	144	156	168	180
Snow shoveling	234	273	312	351	390	429	468	507	546	585
Stair climbing	168	196	224	252	280	308	336	364	392	420
Trimming hedges	126	147	168	189	210	231	252	273	294	315
Vacuuming	90	105	120	135	150	165	180	195	210	225
Washing the car	90	105	120	135	150	165	180	195	210	225
Waxing the car	120	140	160	180	200	220	240	260	280	300
Weeding	120	140	160	180	200	220	240	260	280	300
Window cleaning	90	105	120	135	150	165	180	195	210	225

SEVEN REASONS TO START A PROGRAM OF AEROBIC EXERCISE

Mini-workouts and doing things the hard way will force your body to burn extra calories and help you get used to the idea of being more active. As your body confidence grows, you may want to consider moving on to the next step: a program of regular aerobic exercise. The benefits of such a program are enormous.

To begin with, regular aerobic exercise will help you burn more calories faster, even when you are sitting still. It does this by raising your metabolism—the rate at which your body burns calories—and keeping it elevated for hours after a workout. It also will build muscle while helping to reduce fat, so your body will become firmer and more toned.

There's more. The National Institutes of Health lists these important health benefits:

- Regular physical activity can help prevent heart disease and stroke by strengthening your heart muscle, lowering your blood pressure, raising your high-density lipoprotein (HDL—the "good" cholesterol) levels and lowering your low-density lipoprotein (LDL—the "bad" cholesterol) levels. It also improves blood flow, increasing your heart's working capacity.
- Regular physical activity can reduce blood pressure in people with high blood pressure levels.
- Regular physical activity helps preserve muscle mass during weight loss.
- Regular physical activity helps prevent back pain by increasing muscle strength and endurance and improving flexibility and posture.
- Regular weight-bearing exercise promotes bone formation and helps prevent bone loss associated with aging.
- Regular physical activity can improve your mood and the way you feel about yourself. Researchers also have found that exercise is likely to reduce feelings

of depression and anxiety and can be helpful in managing stress.

PLANNING YOUR PROGRAM

Let's say you're convinced and want to get started with a workout program that offers all the benefits of regular activity. But you're concerned about the consequences of attempting to do too much too soon. The best antidote for this kind of anxiety is to ask your doctor how much and what kind of exercise he or she recommends.

Even if you have full confidence in your physical abilities, get a go-ahead from your doctor before starting an ambitious exercise program if the answer to any of the following questions is yes.

- Do you have heart problems?
- Do you suffer from chest pains?
- Do you often feel faint or have dizzy spells?
- Do you have high blood pressure?
- Do you have bone or joint problems that could be aggravated by exercise?
- Are you over sixty-five and sedentary?
- Are you taking prescription medications, such as those for high blood pressure?
- Is there any other medical reason why you should not engage in a regular exercise program?

Getting Started

Assuming you have your doctor's okay, here's how to plan an exercise program you can live with.

Start by Picking an Easy, Enjoyable Aerobic Activity

Aerobic activities, which involve continuous, rhythmic movement of the large muscles of the body, condition the heart and lungs, accelerate fat loss, and increase muscle mass. This type of exercise also stimulates the body to produce more glucose, serotonin, noradrenaline, and adrenaline, substances that are natural appetite suppressants and mood elevators.

There are many kinds of aerobic activity, and each has advantages and disadvantages. For now, try to narrow your choices down to one or two that you think you'll enjoy doing. Enjoyment will help you stick with it.

Walking, even relatively slow walking, is a great aerobic activity to start with because you can set your own pace, you need no special equipment other than comfortable shoes, you can do it almost anytime, anywhere. And it can be as sociable as you want it to be; with a walking buddy or two, time seems to fly, and the miles pile up unnoticed. Jogging has many of the advantages of walking but is harder on bones and joints.

Swimming is gentler and less stressful to the body than many other aerobic activities, so it is a particularly good choice for people who cannot or should not subject their bones and connective tissue to jolting movements.

Biking and rowing, either outdoors or on stationary machines, provide good aerobic workouts if you have the equipment or belong to a health club.

Other popular aerobic activities to consider if you are in good health include roller skating or in-line skating, aerobic dancing, cross-country skiing, and jumping rope.

Focus on one activity to begin with. Later on, you can incorporate others into your program. Alternating between two or three activities will help prevent boredom (the most often cited reason for giving up on exercise). And because different activities work different muscle groups, alternating allows muscles that are heavily used one day, in one activity, to recoup the next day as you engage in a different activity.

Ease into It

No matter which activity you choose to begin with, it's important to get off to a slow start. Easing into your chosen activity will help prevent stress and strain on underused muscles and will give your heart and lungs a chance to get used to meeting the demands of greater exertion.

A good rule of thumb: If you've been sedentary for the past year, plan to begin with no more than ten minutes of your chosen activity a couple of times a week, and instead of giving it all you've got, keep the pace easy and slow.

Important: Even ten minutes may be too much if you are in very poor condition or if you've chosen a strenuous activity such as rowing or jogging. If your breathing becomes difficult or you feel uncomfortable for any reason, slow down and stop, even if you've only been at it for a minute or two.

Make It Comfortable, and Make It Safe

Wear comfortable, well-fitting shoes that help rather than hinder your performance. The same goes for clothes; you don't have to invest in high-style workout gear, but it is important to wear garments that are absorbent and easy to move in. Don't take chances. If you are going to walk, jog, or bike outdoors, stick to areas that are safe, well patrolled, and well lit. (Many older people feel most comfortable walking in climate-controlled malls where security is good.)

Make It a Habit

Exercise regularly to obtain the greatest fat-burning and health benefits. Try to make it as much a part of your routine as bathing and brushing your teeth. Scheduling workouts for times that suit your biological clock can keep you on track. If you're a morning person, exercise early in the day when you are at your most energetic. If you feel peppiest late in the day, plan activities that can be done in the evening.

Build Up Gradually to Thirty Minutes of Brisk Aerobic Exercise Several Times a Week

Your rate of progress will depend on your age and your starting weight and fitness level, and it may take months before you are able to manage thirty minutes of activity. Never mind. Don't rush it. The idea is to *gradually* increase the frequency, pace, and duration of your workouts, allowing your body time to adjust along the way.

For instance, here's how you might ease into a program of aerobic walking and jogging: On your first few days, start with three or four minutes of easy walking, switch to a brisker pace for another three or four minutes, then back to a more leisurely pace for another three or four minutes. On succeeding days, continue to start at a relaxed pace, but gradually increase the ratio of brisk to easy walking. Once you have worked up to thirty minutes of brisk walking, you might want to add a little jogging to your workout—perhaps thirty seconds or so at first—then switch back to brisk walking for sixty seconds. When that feels comfortable, move up to forty-five seconds of jogging alternating with thirty seconds of brisk walking. And so on. Keep challenging yourself, but do it slowly and sensibly. And give yourself lots of credit for every incremental gain along the way.

WARM UP, CONDITION, COOL DOWN

One of the biggest mistakes made by novice exercisers is to plunge into the conditioning phase of their workout without warming up and to stop cold at the end—a practice that practically invites sore muscles and even injuries. Instead, emulate the pros and divide your workout into distinct stages, beginning with hydration.

1. Prepare for your workout by drinking at least 2 cups water. Do it even if you're not thirsty; starting out fully hydrated will help combat fatigue later on.
2. Take three to five minutes to warm up. Warming up will rev up your circulation and respiration, elevate your body temperature, and get your muscles ready for action, thereby reducing the risk of injury during the more vigorous activity to come. Some people like to warm up with a series of easy calisthenics that

gently work the body's major muscle groups. Others prefer to warm up with an easy, slow version of their workout activity.

3. After your warm-up, begin the "conditioning period"—the phase of activity that increases cardiovascular fitness. Work out at a moderate rate of intensity. Don't knock yourself out. As you continue with regular workouts, gradually you will be able to exercise harder and longer. Increase the conditioning period until you are exercising thirty or more minutes at a time.

   During this conditioning phase, you will notice that you are breathing faster and more deeply and that your heart is beating faster, too. These are all signs that you are challenging your body. Do not challenge yourself to the point of being out of breath. You should be able to carry on a conversation during this phase. If you can't, ease up. You body should recover within a few minutes of your workout and not feel exhausted afterward. Extreme fatigue after exercise is another sign that you are trying too hard and should take it a little easier.

4. Cool off gradually after your workout. Don't come to a dead stop, but instead decrease the intensity of your exercise, then walk around for a few minutes to allow your body to adjust to the decreased physical demands. Finish with a few minutes of stretching to prevent soreness later on.

5. Take another long drink of water (2 cups is the recommended amount) to replenish fluids lost during exercise.

MORE IS BETTER

Exercise physiologists recommend a program that combines aerobic activities with others that build strength (such as weight training) and increase flexibility (stretching, yoga), and at some point you may want to add these to your daily routine. What's most important, however, is not to feel so overwhelmed by all of these recommendations that you do nothing at all. The current thinking on exercise is that more is better (within reason, of course), but that *some* is definitely preferable to none. So do what you can, and keep at it. You'll be glad you did, and that's a promise.

FINAL WORDS

The New Cabbage Soup Diet has put you on the fast track to quick weight loss. You lost a significant number of pounds on your first cycle of the diet. From now on, use the diet periodically to lose more weight more quickly and more easily than you can on any other diet. Just be sure to wait at least fourteen days before resuming the diet. Between cycles, be guided by the Food Guide Pyramid for optimal nutrition, control or maintain your weight with the Cabbage Soup Maintenance Plan, or switch to a slow, safe, long-term diet of your choice for continued weight loss.

As the pounds continue to melt away, incorporate moderate exercise into your life for even easier, more rapid weight loss, better health and fitness, and a greater sense of well-being.

It almost sounds like a prescription for health and happiness, and in many ways, it is. With the New Cabbage Soup Diet as your starting point, and the tips, techniques, and suggestions in this book to help you along, you *can* be healthier and happier.